WHY I GEEK

An Anthology Of Fandom Origin Stories

Edited by
Stephen Webb and Clay Dockery

Coal Hill Press
Boston — Dallas — New York

Published by Coal Hill Press (www.coalhill.com)
Edited by Clay Dockery and Stephen Webb
Cover Artwork and Design by Jennifer Drucker
ISBN: 978-099944790-1

My name is Oliver Queen.
After five years in hell, I returned home with one goal – to save my city.
Today I fight that war on two fronts.
By day, I lead Star City as its Mayor.
But by night, I am someone else.
I am something else.
I am the Green Arrow.*

My name is Stephen Webb.
After 38 years, I decided to achieve one goal – to publish this book.
Today, I dedicate said book to 5 souls.
A.W. for giving me a great life...
C.W. for showing me my purpose...
K.H. for making me believe I can do anything...
C.D. for telling me I wouldn't like it...
& ME, for doing it, despite everything else.
I am the Co-Editor.

My name is Clay Dockery.
I dedicate this book to the incredible people who have shaped my life.
C.E., S.M., A.W., S.G., M.S., S.T., N.K., S.W., K.F., W.D., K.D., and S.S.
... I have failed this format.

Meanwhile, in WHY I GEEK ...

* Oliver Queen was not involved in the creation of this book. We asked him, but he was busy brooding.

TABLE OF CONTENTS

TABLE OF CONTENTS

SPOILER WARNING!

THE NIGHT IS DARK AND FULL OF TERRORS.

Wait...wrong warning...

Spoilers are not limited to the obvious "Kaiser Soze beat Dumbledore with a sled" type reveal, but can also include something as seemingly innocuous as "I'm not going to spoil it, but man you're going to freak out!"

From our perspective, anything that impacts the way you process something for the first time that was planted in your head by someone who had already experienced it should fall under that "spoiler" distinction.

If you are giving this as a way to encourage people to get into your fandom we recommend that you read that section first to make sure you are comfortable with the level of "spoiler" content it may contain.

So that being said:
THIS BOOK CONTAINS SPOILERS.

FOREWORD
by Terry Molloy

Geek   giːk/

noun: **geek**; plural noun: **geeks**

1. an unfashionable or socially inept person.

2. a knowledgeable and obsessive enthusiast.

    "a computer geek"

verb: **geek**; 3rd person present: **geeks**; past tense: **geeked**;

1. engage in or discuss computer-related tasks obsessively or with great attention to technical detail. "We all geeked out for a bit and exchanged ICQ/MSN/AOL/website information"

2. be or become extremely excited or enthusiastic about a subject, typically one of specialist or minority interest. "I am totally geeking out over this upcoming film"

Origin: late 19th century: from the related English dialect word *geck* 'fool', of Germanic origin; related to Dutch *gek* 'mad, silly'.

(Oxford English Dictionary, "geek," accessed September 2, 2017, https://en.oxforddictionaries.com/definition/us/geek.)

In January 1963 I turned 16 years old, a universally recognized age of teenage angst, insecurity, rebellion, and obsession.

I was certainly obsessed with Science Fiction, devouring authors like Isaac Asimov, Arthur C. Clarke, Robert Heinlein, Philip K. Dick, Stanislaw Lem, J. G. Ballard, Kurt Vonnegut, Ray Bradbury, Frank Herbert and John Wyndham with the speed and voracity of a velociraptor.

FOREWORD

In those days you were not a 'Geek' but rather a 'Fan' of a subject... so that when a new TV series called "Doctor Who" first transmitted on the BBC on the 23rd November 1963 (somewhat overshadowed by the assassination of President Kennedy in Dallas the day before) I was front and centre, in prime position both emotionally and intellectually to immerse myself totally in this fascinating and intriguing programme, as an instant 'fan'.

The term 'nerd' or 'geek' didn't really surface in common usage until the dawning of the computer age and was mainly reserved for those whose obsession was for the more esoteric reaches of computer programming that excluded the 'ordinary' person, though this spread rapidly to encompass those with any sort of obsession. Geeks were considered loners, socially awkward, with a driving desire for the minutiae of a particular subject.

Nowadays being referred to as a 'Geek' has morphed into a more general term for those addicted or driven by their love of particular TV programmes (normally Sci-Fi), range of books, comics or films.... a badge of courage and pride for the wearer as social media has enabled the 'geeks' to realize that they are not alone hiding in a dark cupboard with their fantastical beliefs, but there are many more, just like them, out there.

I'm definitely a Geek; you probably are too if you are reading this excellent book "Why I Geek..." containing 'confessions' from 'Geeks' of all genres. So, Geeks of the Universe...Unite! You have nothing to lose but your sanity.... as you try to work out how your animatronic cosplay costume for 'Cthulhu' can ever be realistically created at less than 70 feet high!

Enjoy this lovely book and... "May the 'Geek' be with you"...

—Terry Molloy, 2017

INTRODUCTION
by Stephen Webb and Clay Dockery

A not so long time ago in a school hallway not far far away, being a "geek" or a "nerd" was the same as being an outcast. It meant being shunted aside or bullied. It meant that your loves and obsessions were something to hide, not something to stand tall behind. To be fair – times have changed. We are no longer seen as the locker stuffed, pocket protector wearing stereotypes that so many 80s movies portrayed us to be. The geeks have inherited the earth. Science Fiction, fantasy, role-playing games, comics, even statistical analysis in sports; all of the things that any of us in our late 30s or older had to fight to talk about in public have become mainstream. As a result, our focus has changed from trying to defend our geekdom itself to trying to defend the sheer amount of time, energy, money, and emotional resources that we allocate to the things we love.

Instead of being stuffed in a locker it is far more likely that you have heard something like, "I mean, sure... I like *comics* as much as the next person, but I just don't get how you can spend so much time talking about it." If you're an enthusiastic, committed, and driven fan of any particular fandom then you have probably heard those words repeatedly, and perhaps from friends or loved ones. If you're not the sort of fan who goes all in, it is possible that you may have been the one who said the words to your own friends or family – even if it was just to your "misguided" coworker who obsesses over *Star Trek* conventions. You may even be familiar with the well-meaning (but exceedingly annoying) statement, *"Imagine if you put all of that energy you spend on Doctor Who into something that matters."*

Introduction

And who could forget getting pulled into that uncomfortable conversation with your uncle at Thanksgiving who seemingly tries to connect with everyone but just shakes his head when you mention that your latest batch of action figures have arrived. If you didn't at least furrow your brow and crinkle your nose because you've experienced something similar to these scenarios then consider yourself very lucky.

For many of us, it is difficult to explain to people who aren't into these geeky pursuits why it is that we love what we love. The first step is not to define "fan" or "fandom"; these aren't answers that are going to come from a dictionary. This entire process is far more visceral than that. Being a fan... a "fanatic", or really in today's terminology being a "geek", is rooted in an emotional reaction to the given material. In most cases becoming a truly invested geek also includes a desire to learn and consume more about the topic. At a certain point, the nature of fandom overwhelms both the logical and emotional parts of your brain, and in that moment you become a "superfan".

Once you have crossed that moment you can better understand the appeal of attending the big fan conventions. When you are at the convention, it feels like those family vacations you took as a kid where the destination was familiar and you could be at ease and just... belong. You are in a building full of people, most of whom are not a part of your particular fandom, but who absolutely understand how rewarding it can be to be unapologetically passionate about a topic that the majority of society would likely define as "trivial".

Once we hit upon this concept, we decided it would be fun and interesting to work on a project that would help people express these ideas

Introduction

about fandom to others. Just between the two of us we have an enormous range of interests: we have a podcast about Doctor Who, work on a Harry Potter convention, collect and display a large amount of rare and valuable items, attend Star Wars events regularly, and so on. So the basic idea of this book was formed. We knew we wanted to focus on trying to bridge the awkward gap between fans and family – if for no other reason than to make those holiday dinners a little less awkward.

At what seemed like the 400th discussion about our fandoms and interests and how we wanted to approach this project, we had that lightbulb moment. No matter what the subject, everyone has an entry point, or origin story, to their fandom, and everyone has a story that deserves to be heard. While each person, in each fandom, is unique, the core concept of what fandom means is rooted in a similar set of experiences. In our travels to various conventions, meetups, and events we've gotten to know a great number of smart and creative people of many different backgrounds who are interested in different but interconnected things all in the name of fandom. We considered the people we know whose primary fandom may be different from ours as well as those who also love the same things we do, but do so from their own unique perspectives. We decided it would be essential to include voices and lenses other than our own.

In order to make this happen, we discussed a wide variety of topics and potential contributors. We threw out dozens of ideas before ultimately narrowing it down to those included in this volume. (We already have a list of many additional fandoms, contributors, and stories out there just waiting to be told in future volumes!) The scope of what could be considered a "fandom" in this collection is intentionally wide. The topics we ultimately chose to make a part of this anthology include not just the obviously "geeky" fandoms" like *Star Trek* and *Doctor Who* but also fandoms that may not usually be thought of with that terminology, like the *West Wing* and pro-wrestling. It is not typical for stories of music fandom, "prestige TV shows", or sports to make their way into a book aimed at "geeks" but we believe that the stories speak for themselves. Our essential point is simple: these ways to experience fandom are not altogether different. In fact, you may even find that the differences between fantasy sports and Dungeons & Dragons players are simply trading a jersey number for a sigil.

No matter what it is that we love, or how we express the love of it, it is the collective experience of sharing and reveling in that fandom that can draw us all closer together. As we read each individual origin story it became evident that a common theme in fandom is finding a place of belonging. That place, whether it is discovered in the cockpit of the Millennium Falcon, the stands of a baseball stadium, or the pages of a comic book is where we first find the comfort that allows us to not only be ourselves but to be with others – unguarded and unapologetic.

Once we had all of those ideas together, they quickly developed into the collection of essays that became *Why I Geek: An Anthology of Fandom Origin Stories*. Every tale has a beginning, every hero has an origin, and every fan has a story of how and why they developed their connection to their particular fandom. Just as each fandom is unique, so too is each essay in this anthology. Some are personal and emotional, others are straightforward and academic, and still others may be an electric dream state that traverses the rules of time... and prose. Each has been written in the unique voice and perspective of the author, and we have intentionally left in dialectical

Introduction

spellings and colloquialisms. Yet each and every essay gives an essential insight into why we are fans and what is compelling about the nature of being fans.

It seems as though, no matter what fandoms we are a part of, every day there is another franchise-defining blockbuster, every week there is a convention, every minute there is something new and specific to that fandom that draws in new fans and means there is a new type of experience for the existing fans. This overwhelming cacophony of material can sometimes make it seem like the connections being made are less meaningful, as there is just too much to experience fully. The following collection of essays should also show that this is not the case. This anthology represents the many ways that we all have developed very deep and personal connections to the things we love, and it attempts to give a small insight into the ways in which, no matter what we love, our stories are interconnected.

These stories are not about what it means to be a fan in a tangible sense, nor histories of how fandoms of certain things came to be. These are personal connections, the reflections of individuals in particular moments. These are just some examples of the intense ways that the fandoms built on the foundation of those worlds have created communities, fictional and very real, that continue to bind and connect people. Our experiences of the world are rooted in our identity, the lenses through which we see things, and the lenses through which others see us. For most of us, deep down, we want nothing more than to be understood, to be accepted and sometimes to be exalted. The ways we see ourselves and the ways we can express who we are take many forms: we may band together over a shared experience, a shared

Introduction

belief, or a shared love. Within any given world that love may be expressed with writing fan fiction, or cosplaying, or presenting at conventions, or cheering when your favorite character made it through the *Game of Thrones* finale, or any number of other ways to express what we love.

These are stories of sharing that love. While these are examples from just a few fandoms, there are thousands of additional worlds to explore and millions of stories to tell within each. We hope this volume will serve as an introduction and a call for people to allow themselves to be open to these experiences. We hope that when the question arises (as it inevitably will), "why do you care so much about that?" a geek in any fandom can hand over this book and say, "because it makes me feel like this."

We hope these stories move you like they moved us, and that you all continue to express yourselves in powerful and unique ways. These are stories of people's connections to shared passions, and hopefully a call for all of us to connect more, to advocate for change, to love freely and openly, and to stand firm for the important things we hold dear.

We hope you enjoy it and that together we can each tell our continued stories of "Why I Geek".

DOCTOR WHO
"Why You Should Never Give an Academic a Time Machine"
by Robert Smith?

TARDIS materialisation circuit: Sydney, June 12, 1978.

It was the giant fly that did it.

This story begins in 1978, in June, in Sydney, Australia. I'm almost six years old and damn was I busy. You see, I absolutely loved TV and I'd made very serious commitments to my shows. Monday was *Mr. Squiggle*, about a spacefaring puppet who lived on the moon and came to earth to draw upside-down pictures. Exciting! Tuesday was *Flipper*, a water-based version of Lassie but with a dolphin who somehow still rescued Timmy from the mine shaft by squeaking. Riveting! Wednesday was *Humphrey B Bear*, about a giant, silent bear who... Hey, don't judge me; it was Australia, and we only had two channels. That sort of thing passed for entertainment back then.

On this particular June day, I was making some model aeroplanes in my bedroom when I decided to wander into the living room to see what my family was watching. It was a moment that was to change the destiny of millions.

vworp vworp

TARDIS materialisation circuit: various times. Circa 1950s and 1960s

Only this story doesn't really begin in 1978. It began decades earlier than that, because my father had been a big fan of William Hartnell. He'd loved everything the actor had been in, watching all his movies and television appearances. Including a little TV show called *Doctor Who*.

Robert Smith?

My dad hadn't really been a fan of the show per se, just a fan of the man who'd played the first Doctor. Which means my father, a non-fan, has seen episodes that were since wiped from the archives. (The BBC deleted a bunch of episodes in the seventies because they couldn't imagine anyone ever wanting to watch *Doctor Who* again. Yes, really.) My father has seen episodes I'll never get to see. I quizzed him about this once, but he doesn't remember them. Sigh. My own flesh and blood.

vworp vworp

TARDIS materialisation circuit: fast return to 1978

So, in 1978, my father is watching *Doctor Who* for old times' sake. William Hartnell is no longer the Doctor; the episode in question is *The Green Death*, starring Jon Pertwee. In fact, Pertwee wasn't even the current Doctor at that time, but Australia was awash with repeats of *Doctor Who* even then. So much for the BBC's idea that nobody would want to watch the show more than once. Maybe they just hated Australians?

I'm watching the climactic episode of this story, starring a flamboyant scientist, a bunch of soldiers running around and giant maggots. Giant. Maggots. This is amazing. The maggots are overwhelming the countryside, with the soldiers unable to stop them.

I decide to return to my room.

Not because what I was watching was bad. Far from it. But, you see, I was busy. My TV schedule was full, and I just couldn't commit to another show. It wasn't easy being a five-year-old Australian kid, but I had priorities, dammit.

So I'm back in my room, working hard on my paper aeroplanes. I take my work very seriously. But I reach a natural stopping point and think that maybe, just maybe, I might go back to the living room. Just to see.

I'm standing in the doorway, watching half-interestedly. By this point, the flamboyant scientist has cooked up an antidote to the giant maggots and is driving a yellow sports car around the countryside, tossing food out. This was pretty good stuff, but I wasn't going to be swayed. I had commitments.

And then I saw it.

I saw the most beautiful and the most terrifying thing I'd ever laid eyes on. A giant fly, the end result of the same mutation that had caused the maggots to grow. A giant fly.

A. Giant. Fly.

It was astonishing. I stared open-mouthed from that doorway as the Doctor battled that giant fly with his cape, the monster dive-bombing him. It was thrilling. It was frightening. It was the most incredible thing my five-year-old eyes had ever seen. I was utterly hooked.

TARDIS materialisation circuit: the mid-nineties and onwards

Never mind that the giant fly is now seen as an embarrassing failure of special effects and bad editing, something to be laughed over. Never mind that the third Doctor, once seen as a benign mother hen, is now seen as a patriarchal Tory selling out his pacifist ways to cozy up with the military. Never mind that we now know the giant maggots were actually condoms and thus none of us can ever unsee that whenever we re-watch the episode. Never mind that we grew up and came to mock the very thing we loved. Never mind all that.

vworp vworp

3

Robert Smith?

TARDIS materialisation circuit: Sydney, 1978

Despite my busy schedule, somehow I made time for this new show. I had to. The very next night I sat down to watch Episode 1 of *The Time Warrior*. I met Sarah Jane Smith, who would be the Doctor's longest-serving companion...

vworp vworp

TARDIS materialisation circuit: Illinois, 2006

— and who would eventually turn up in the new series alongside David Tennant, inextricably linking —

vworp vworp

TARDIS materialisation circuit: June 13, 1978

...my childhood to...

vworp vworp

TARDIS materialisation circuit: North America, 2006+

...my adulthood on the other side of the world.

vworp vworp

The Australian Broadcasting Corporation showed a single half-hour episode every night at 6:30, so meals had to be scheduled around it (family rules dictated that we could not watch TV over dinner, under any circumstances). I turned my brother into something of a fan and was delighted to discover my much older cousin was already one.

I wasn't particularly wowed by the TARDIS, the Doctor's time machine that looked like a police box on the outside and a futuristic space centre on the inside. It wasn't even in the first episode I watched. But I was taken by the Doctor himself: he was brilliant, funny, flamboyant and confident. Everything I wanted to be. With one obvious exception, the brilliance, although that was the only quality I actually possessed back then, much to my disappointment.

My father and I never bonded over this show once the generational torch had been passed. Despite having been the catalyst, he thought it was all a bit silly and didn't appreciate my newfound obsession with it. I guess the fact that William Hartnell wasn't the star anymore was pretty crushing for him.

vworp vworp

TARDIS materialisation circuit: 24 January, 1980

Though there was that one time, when they showed *The Brain of Morbius* in omnibus form late one night. It was too violent to be shown at 6:30, so they'd screened the entire four-part story after my bedtime. My father casually mentioned this the next day, so I grilled him and grilled him as to its contents, but he'd only caught the tail end of it. I still wanted to know everything I could. He was no help.

vworp vworp

TARDIS materialisation circuit: 1980–1988.

My friends and I play *Doctor Who* every lunchtime in the playground. At first we use a tree for the TARDIS, but once we get to high school we use a stairwell, which seems much more fitting. None of us are in the cool group, because during those years you have to be a nerd to watch *Doctor Who*, so we're all outcasts and misfits. Some, I later discover, are gay (though that would never have been admitted in the playground). Some are nerds. Some are just plain weird. We bonded together for the simple fact that no one else would have us.

I'm always the Doctor, partly because I'm the biggest fan (though everyone watches religiously) and partly because I'm the smartest.

That's not a boast. Being smart was in no way a desirable quality back then, even among nerds. It was my curse. But the fact that the Doctor was also the smartest person in the room made it just a little bit easier. Maybe I could embrace that like he did...?

vworp vworp

TARDIS materialisation circuit: Ottawa, May 2015

I'm standing before an applauding crowd, being handed a incredibly prestigious award in the nation's capital. I'm an actual ambassador! Of mathematics, it's true, but an ambassador nonetheless. For my abilities to reach out to the world and make the discipline internationally recognisable. This award will look great next to my Guinness World Record. What nobody realises is that I have *Doctor Who* to thank for both of these things.

vworp vworp

TARDIS materialisation circuit: January, 1989

I'm 16 years old, and I've been a *Doctor Who* fan for as long as I can remember. But I'm shaking in my boots. Because I'm on my way to my very first *Doctor Who* event. Aside from my high-school friends — we don't play *Doctor Who* anymore, because we're desperate to be grownups now, but we do still talk about it — I've never met another truly hardcore fan before. And now I'm going to a *Doctor Who* party. Where there will be fans everywhere. What if I don't know as much as they do? What if they quiz me and find me lacking? Will there be any girls there?

None of my fears come to pass. Actually, no one really speaks to me, because it's not that kind of a party. Mostly, we sit in a university lecture hall and watch the latest episodes that someone has copied from a copy of someone's VHS tape from Britain. I'm fine with that. I'm watching the latest episode months before it'll show on the ABC. I even get to watch some older episodes, in black and white. The kind that never get shown on the ABC. This is pretty awesome.

And no, there were no girls there. Well, there were a few older women, one Kate Orman among them, but nobody my age. I'm not sure whether to be relieved or disappointed.

vworp vworp

TARDIS materialisation circuit: December 1991

I'm a disaffected 19 year old who's just given up on his social group. I decided I was being too complacent by having friends and the like, so I walked out on everybody, vowing to make it on my own. What could possibly go wrong...?

vworp vworp

TARDIS materialisation circuit: February 1992

Three months later and I'm miserable. I have no friends and nothing to do. I see an ad in the latest Doctor Who fan club newsletter looking for volunteers. They need people who can fold the newsletter and stuff them into envelopes. It really was a different time. The reward was only that you'd get to see snippets that no one else would. I signed up, more out of boredom than anything else.

At the first folding meeting, held in someone's living room on a Friday night, there are six of us, folding 300 newsletters in thirds and putting them in envelopes. It's dull work, but we get to watch recently discovered episodes of *The Ice Warriors*, a 1967 story I'd never seen. That's pretty amazing. As we watch and fold and fold some more, we get to chatting. The jokes flow easily, because we have a common language.

The next day, we meet at a different house and do it all again. And then again the day after. Some of the people go to all three folding events of the weekend, some only one or two. But it's a much more intimate crowd than the parties. There is a girl there, Sarah, who seems quite nice...

vworp vworp

TARDIS materialisation circuit: October 1992

... I discover that my friend Sarah, whom I've become quite close to and have been mildly crushing on, is in fact a lesbian. I'm shocked, because I had no idea. I'm even more shocked because she came out via a fan newsletter, announcing it to the world — or at least the *Doctor Who* fan world. I've never met a lesbian before, at least as far as I know. The world is clearly much bigger than I've imagined.

vworp vworp

TARDIS materialisation circuit: July 1992

I attend my first convention. It's an overnight event, so I'm staying in my first hotel. I have two random roommates... one of whom I never meet, because he spends the entire night in the video room watching episodes. I've made a few friends through the folding meetings, I make a few more at the convention, and my cousin turns up, so suddenly there's critical mass of people to talk to. Six of us stand around talking, nodding hello to Dallas, the organiser, as he walks past...

... and several hours later, Dallas walks by again, saying "You guys haven't moved for the past three hours!"

Someone came up with a theory that the reason it's so easy to make friends in the fan community is because the most embarrassing thing about you is actually the reason you're there in the first place. Which means you can kind of relax and let go. Works for me.

vworp vworp

TARDIS materialisation circuit: December 1989

Did I mention that the show finished airing new episodes some years earlier? It didn't really slow us down. One of the great appeals of *Doctor Who* is that there's simply so much of it, so we spent years catching up on episodes we missed, trading video tapes across the world. And we got thoughtful too: the fan newsletter stopped being about the latest news and started becoming analytical, delving deep into the themes and structures of old episodes.

This meant you'd have to go back and watch them all over again in order to appreciate the new insights. Well, if we have to, we have to. And I had some analytical insights of my own along the way. I decided that I should write some of those down.

vworp vworp

TARDIS materialisation circuit: July 1993

It's my second convention, and I'm volunteering to help out behind the scenes. I get to meet the guests, which is pretty cool. I bond with actresses Mary Tamm and Katy Manning (who played companions to the third and fourth Doctors) over dinner, because they're also vegetarians. I participate in the con itself, but I find that it's the friends I'm making that are the most meaningful.

vworp vworp

TARDIS materialisation circuit: December 1993

Kate Orman has taken over as president of the fan club. She decides to decentralise the structure and create sub-groups. I've volunteered to create one, without any idea of what to do. She puts me in touch with Neil, who was thinking much the same thing but is a lot better organised. He takes me on as his second-in-command. And incidentally offers me a job. By this point, I've finished my degree in science, majoring in mathematics.

Oh, and I find myself a girlfriend as well. And she hates *Doctor Who*. D'oh.

vworp vworp

TARDIS materialisation circuit: March 1991

I decide to major mathematics when at university, but why? For that we need to travel back a decade...

vworp vworp

TARDIS materialisation circuit: 1981

... to a 1981 *Doctor Who* story called *Logopolis*. It was Tom Baker's final story as the Doctor and featured a team of mathematicians holding the universe together. Through mathematics, they control the basic building blocks of everything.

"Structure is the essence of matter," says the lead mathematician in that story, "And the essence of matter is mathematics." Truer words have never been spoken. As a fairly gifted child, I could have gone in any number of directions. But it was *Doctor Who* — and *Logopolis* in particular — that set me on my path. With its emphasis on recursion, hexadecimal code and numbers maintaining the universe, *Logopolis* fascinated me and drove me to study mathematics.

In essence, you can whittle anything down to mathematics. Earthquakes, tsunamis, disease, marriage, a conversation... they can all be expressed by mathematics, and the logic of analysis can be used to understand and predict the future. Mathematics is probably the most powerful thing human beings have ever invented.

Logopolis gets this and makes it meaningful. Block Transfer Computation — creating solid objects via the power of muttering numbers — may not seem that scientifically likely, but it's a useful metaphor for just how powerful mathematics can be. Because what mathematics does is take chaos and turn it into order. When the mathematicians fail in *Logopolis*, the entire universe is threatened with destruction from the chaos.

vworp vworp

TARDIS materialisation circuit: 1994

My honours thesis is in chaos theory. I study a new type of chaotic behaviour, called superchaos, that might well predict the end of all life as we know it. I'm sure that's just a coincidence.

vworp vworp

TARDIS materialisation circuit: March 1991

The message of *Logopolis* is clear: mathematics is all. From the sweep of history to the prediction of the future, mathematics is the essence of everything around us. Understand mathematics well enough and you can pretty much do anything. Challenge accepted.

vworp vworp

TARDIS materialisation circuit: July 1991

Kate Orman happened to be the librarian at the university where I'm studying. I nervously introduce myself to her one day and we have an awkward conversation, as though we shouldn't really be talking about our secret life in the wider world.

In the *Doctor Who* newsletter, she writes about vegetarianism. It gets me thinking.

In the university newspaper, she writes about feminism. It gets me thinking.

vworp vworp

TARDIS materialisation circuit: January 1992

I'm now a committed vegetarian and a committed feminist. The world has gotten so much bigger than I could have imagined, and my mind is more open than I ever thought possible. Thanks to *Doctor Who*, my guiding lights have become compassion and kindness.

vworp vworp

TARDIS materialisation circuit: January 1994

Neil's job doesn't last long, but the club does. We assemble in an echoey church hall in the middle of nowhere to watch old *Doctor Who* and new *Star Trek: The Next Generation*. Meanwhile, Kate Orman publishes her first novel, in the *Doctor Who: The New Adventures* line. These books have become the only fix of new *Who* since the show went off the air, so she's basically become a rock star in the *Doctor Who* world.

I watch how she acts with her newfound fame — she's hilarious and makes everyone laugh — and think "I could do that."

vworp vworp

TARDIS materialisation circuit: August 2009

My students and I write a comedy academic article on mathematical modelling of zombies as a disease. My students weren't sure their professor would go for it, but they didn't realise I had science fiction in my blood. I decide to publish it, mainly to amuse myself.

The zombie article goes viral in the media. My phone rings off the hook: BBC News, the Wall Street Journal, you name it. For 24 hours, it was the Number 1 story in the world (it was a slow news month). I get invited to do TV, radio and go on the lecture circuit, where I'm described as the most famous living mathematician. I'm even flown to Hollywood, where I participate in a panel with George Romero and Max Brooks as part of the Hollywood Science and Entertainment Exchange. I get into an argument with George Romero about the nature of zombies.

My students and I even win a Guinness World Record for the first-ever mathematical model of a zombie invasion. It's one of the lesser Guinnesses, but on the bright side no one can supersede it. I'll take it.

Throughout it all, I find that the key is maintaining the humour. I revel in the irony of what's happening, and the jokes sustain themselves, partly because I'm an actual professor but partly because I just inherently "get" the nature of genre fiction and its effect on the masses.

vworp vworp

TARDIS materialisation circuit: August 1995

With a bachelor's and an honour's degree in mathematics under my belt, I'm leaving Australia. I've been accepted into the Ph.D. program at McMaster University in Canada, so once again I'm leaving everyone behind. I throw a giant party, which people from all walks of my life attend. With such a diverse bunch, the only common fact they'll all know about me is my love of Doctor Who. So I make a speech and end it by transforming my regular look into the sixth Doctor's coat of many colours, announcing that I'm going to become "a colourful Canadian identity".

Kate Orman, Neil, Dallas, Sarah and other fan friends are there to see me off. Kate incidentally mentions that I should go to the Chicago convention in November, as she'll be flying across the world to attend it.

VORTEX CRUNCH

TARDIS materialisation circuit, hard landing: Hamilton, Canada, September 1995. Regeneration in progress.

I'm in a new hemisphere, and everything is upside down. I know nobody. I've never lived away from home before. I don't even know how to do laundry. (I learn this the hard way when I put the whites in with the colours and turn all my shirts pink.) I'm in a massive culture-shock meltdown

But there's one thing that saves me: *Doctor Who*. Not the show, which is long over, but the fandom. There's an online group called rec.arts.drwho, which I join. From there, I connect with random fans in Canada and all over the world and discover that we can have exactly the same conversations as I had with fans in Australia. Only now I can have them every day, instead of just at monthly meetups. This island of consistency is exactly what I need.

vworp vworp

TARDIS materialisation circuit: November 1995

I take a long train journey from Toronto to Chicago with two fans, in order to attend the Chicago convention. Despite never having met before, we don't run out of conversation in the slightest. For ten hours straight. One of my travelling companions is Graeme Burk...

vworp vworp

Doctor Who

TARDIS materialisation circuit: 2012

My co-author Graeme and I have just won an award for our latest book, *Who Is The Doctor*, an episode guide to the New Series of *Doctor Who*. It's also been endorsed by Neil Gaiman and sold out of its first print run. The rejuvenated version of the show is riding high in the ratings, and we're surfing that wave to fan stardom. We couldn't be happier.

vworp vworp

TARDIS materialisation circuit: December 1997

...the other travelling companion becomes my second lover, in a whirlwind affair before she leaves the country forever. That's quite the train ride.

vworp vworp

TARDIS materialisation circuit: Chicago, November 1995

I have such an amazing time at the Chicago convention. Kate Orman meets her future husband, Jon Blum, there; they've been chatting online, but he lives in Maryland, so they're an early example of an international internet romance. I know Jon independently from rec.arts.drwho, and I happen to run into them in the hotel lobby as they arrive in the shuttle from the airport, having just met. I'm excitedly talking to them, happy that two people I know from opposite sides of the world are here in my life.

They look at me awkwardly. I look back in puzzlement.

They look at me awkwardly again.

We're in a hotel.

They've. Just. Met.

Uh, I'll give them some privacy...

vworp vworp

Robert Smith?

TARDIS materialisation circuit: All future years

Conventions become a mainstay of my life. They're like giant parties, where everyone attends, many in costume. I've also cosplayed, dressing as the sixth and seventh Doctors on occasion. Nobody judges you for this strange thing, because everyone's doing their own strange thing. There are panels to go to, guests giving presentations, room parties, dances, karaoke...

I make friends and lovers. Meanwhile, my career takes me on postdoctoral fellowships to London, Ontario; Los Angeles; Champaign, Illinois; and then back to Canada for a professorship at the University of Ottawa. This chaos is deeply unsettling, but the *Doctor Who* world remains my island of stability.

The show returns to TV in 2005. I adore it from the first minute. I introduce others to it, including my current girlfriend, who comes to love it (phew). I discover that people from all walks of life watch it and self-identify as a fan. Which is no longer a dirty word.

I write books about *Doctor Who*, about zombies and about mathematics. I become a guest at the conventions, signing books and appearing on stage and on panels. I hang out in the green room with the actors. I become genuine friends with Andrew Cartmel, the script editor from the eighties, who writes an introduction to my latest zombie book. I pay my good fortune forward, recruiting other fans to be published in books I'm editing, many for the first time.

But I find it's the friendships I've made that really matter. That's what keeps me coming back again and again. The show is the skeleton around which these connections are built. It's like the weather: endlessly discussable — and if you don't like it now, something new will be along shortly.

Doctor Who

I become a world-leading expert in mathematical modelling of infectious diseases. My work on HPV vaccination causes the policy to be changed in Canada. My work on adherence to HIV medications allows me to calculate the number of doses that can be safely missed before the virus mutates. My work on spraying insecticide to combat malaria in Africa determines better ways to plan the interventions — and shows how the strategy can be updated to account for climate change. I publish the first-ever mathematical model on Guinea-Worm Disease, identifying education as the key component to eradicating this ancient scourge. These and other projects contribute to countless lives being saved. And it would never have happened without a silly little TV show about a flamboyant scientist fighting evil. Only now I'm the flamboyant scientist fighting evil.

vworp vworp

TARDIS materialisation circuit: Present day

I'm a tenured professor, crisscrossing the world in the course of my research. I find myself in random cities for work and often look up *Doctor Who* friends, who are scattered all over. I return to Australia every year, finding that my other friends have all dissipated and are no longer independently friends with each other, but the *Doctor Who* networks are strong. I catch up with Dallas, Neil, Sarah, Kate Orman, Jon Blum and others while I'm there. Graeme Burk and I continue to write books together and even take the occasional long train ride, where we still talk for hours nonstop. We don't always talk about the thing that brought us together, because we're genuine friends now, but it's never far from our minds either.

Doctor Who is the one constant in my life. It's informed so many of my choices and sent me in directions I would never have imagined. I'm a better person because of it. The nonviolent, science-based, compassionate ethos of the show have informed every fibre of my being, making me someone I genuinely like. And the world of fandom is full of interesting people. Some are weird, some are gay, some are misfits, some are outcasts, and some are nerds. In fact, it's not so different to my high-school friends, all those years ago, although it's a lot more socially acceptable now. The maggots have learned how to fly.

The more things change, the more *Doctor Who* stays the same. I'll be a fan until the day I die.

vworp vworp

TARDIS materialisation circuit: June 12, 1978

I'm five years old and there's a giant fly on my TV screen. This is the greatest thing I've ever seen. Even at this young age, I realise the magnitude of what I'm watching. Everything is going to change from this moment on. My entire life has just irrevocably altered course.

Seeing that fly made all the difference. Both to myself and, it turned out, a great many people throughout the world. I went in as a boy... and came out a fan.

STAR WARS
"Carrie On!"
by Christine Evans

My first real memory as a person is of Star Wars. The memory is not just images or feelings, but actual thoughts and a sequence of events. I was almost five and those memories would shape my whole life. In a couple months, I would start kindergarten. In a couple weeks, I would accidentally put my arm through a window (an event causing major trauma, leading to surgery and a lifelong fear of needles). But most vividly of all, I remember the ride home after seeing Star Wars.

Do children really understand how movies work? I know I didn't. My memory of that night isn't of the movie itself but is of my family heading home after leaving the theatre. My parents owned a 1975 blue LTD Ford – a huge beast of a car, a true land cruiser. As we got in the car to make the thirty minute journey home from the Four Seasons Resort Cinema, the only theater within an hour of our small town to be playing Star Wars, I took my place in my favorite seat, the back window. How's that for child safety? From that dangerous and unstable spot I was able to lie flat and look up out at the night sky through the back window of the car. It was magical; all I could see was the stars.

At that moment I chose to believe that the movie screen was just a giant intergalactic picture frame and the characters were just on the other side of the wall, acting their story out. I definitely did not understand how movies worked and so I had this thought as the explanation of what I had just seen, because as I lay there, stretched out head to toe in the back window of this land cruiser, I was looking for them.

Han, Luke, Chewie and Leia were all real, especially Leia. They were out there, somewhere. And if I looked at the stars long enough and hard enough I would be able to see the Millennium Falcon streaking away, taking them off on their next adventure. I genuinely looked for them, muttering under my breath, "they're out there, they're out there." And then another thought came to me, one that will forever be burned into my mind, "She was so pretty, please God, when I grow up, please let me look like Princess Leia."

I had no idea then that Princess Leia was a real woman, a 19 year old daughter of Hollywood royalty named Carrie Fisher. I just knew that Princess Leia Organa was feisty, and beautiful, and awesome, and I wanted nothing more than to be her and look like her. I believe we are granted one pure wish in our lifetimes... and I had just spent mine.

My love of Star Wars survived long beyond that car ride home – like most kids at that time it was everything to me. My folks didn't have a lot of money, so I wasn't collecting the toys in the cool Darth Vader shaped action figure tote – it was the neighbors who had that experience. But my parents did get me books. And with those books and a crazy vivid imagination I spent the days playing Star Wars. I, of course, was Leia. Luke was always one of my imaginary friends, and in fact he was a great imaginary friend (a fact I would later pass along to Mark Hamill himself). My little brother was still too young to play with, and my imagination and need to be world-building didn't make me many friends. But I always had Luke.

Oh, and there was also Han (also imaginary). But imaginary Han wasn't allowed off of the swing set: he kept trying to be "in charge" and this little Princess was having none of that. If you have met me, you know I haven't changed much – I do like my "rogues" but I definitely blame most of my take charge attitude on our fiery space princess.

As time passed, other obsessions took hold: *Thundercats, Elfquest,* boys, *The Dark Crystal, Star Trek,* and *The Phantom of the Opera.* My interests changed, but if *Star Wars* was ever on, I was there to watch it. About the same time that I got my first job I started hearing IT. As I shoveled overpriced popcorn and candy bars at people, they would look back at the girl handing them their change and ask, "Do you know who you look like?" As a salty teenager (pun intended) this didn't thrill me, grand wish of a five year old or not. I was my own person, not a reproduction of some space actress; or was I?

I will never forget sitting in front of the TV one afternoon soon after I got Star Wars on VHS. I turned the box over and there she was. The picture is a side view of Carrie Fisher illuminated by a green light as she bends over the map schematic during the battle of Yavin. Any time I look at it, I can almost hear the words from the movie in my ears, "the Death Star approaching, Death Star will be in range in two minutes." But at that moment I had made a bigger discovery: all of those irritating people were right. I had gotten my wish. I looked just like Princess Leia.

High School and college were a blur of costumes and fandoms, mostly Victorian. Despite constantly working on costumes I hadn't made any that were remotely sci-fi related until the Star Wars Special Edition came out. I guess by that point I had held my continued Star Wars fandom as my little secret until I could find friends to share it with. The Special Editions though, they were the start of something new. Star Wars was in theatres again and there was even talk of more NEW movies. I had to be a part of this.

Using skills built up over years of historical clothing construction, I obsessed over fabric for my first Princess Leia costume, which was the classic Senatorial gown from *A New Hope*. I spray painted boots, found a silver belt, and finally, the crowning glory – the space buns. The first time I ever wore it was for Halloween at the bookstore where I worked. I can't even remember if I asked my boss if it was okay or not. I went in to work all "bunned up" and went about my day. I would be lying if I told you I didn't hold "the pose" a little as I bent over re-shelving mass market paperbacks. Customers would walk past the aisle I was in, stop, back up, and look down the aisle at me, with jaws hanging. In my head I thought, "I could get used to this." I even had regulars come back in later after their initial visits with a camera or to haul a friend in to see me in person. It was exciting. I felt like a Princess.

The second worst date I ever went on was to the Special Edition release of *Return of the Jedi*. (The worst date I ever went on is a story for another time.) The random guy who walked into the theatre dressed up as Luke was more interesting than my date.

The first time I ever called in "sick" to work was for the release of *The Phantom Menace*. I went to wait in line all day and I was dressed up. I got pulled to the front of the line, given free pizza and interviewed for a local radio station. A note to the wise: it doesn't matter if you change your name, if the DJ is going on and on about how much you look like a certain universally recognizable actor, you better hope that your boss isn't listening. The next day at work I had to buy every copy of the area newspaper because my picture was in it. This can be a significant drawback if you work in a book store. However, if my boss knew what I had done, he must have been a secret member of the Rebel Alliance because I still had a job.

Star Wars

I wore the costume a few more times, but that was before fandom conventions or cosplay had developed into such a normal thing, especially in my area of the country, so the buns were put into retirement and the dress packed away and stored.

Years passed and I lived another life. I moved to New York City to pursue an acting career. As my collection of fandoms continued to increase, I added Harry Potter and a growing love of Doctor Who to the mix and started making costumes and finding friends in those worlds. Eventually, I landed a job as a "Sorter" for the traveling exhibit of the Magic of Harry Potter. In that job, I was chosen to attend a children's event on the USS Intrepid Sea Air and Space Museum. It was while there on that ship docked in the Hudson River that I would encounter the Rebel Legion.

The Rebel Legion is a Lucasfilm (and now Disney) recognized, charity based, Star Wars Costume group. These folks know how to make a pretty costume! As I stood there in my wizarding robes with my sassy talking sorting hat I got to meet Luke (this one not even imaginary!), R2-D2, and a beautiful redheaded Jedi that I just decided had to be Mara Jade (I had read all the books and I thought I knew everything!). Anyway, after talking to this great group of people with my adorable British accent that would have even impressed grand Moff Tarkin himself, I sorted Luke into Gryffindor, and R2 into Hufflepuff (I will defend this decision to the grave). I then noticed that the "Mara" Jedi had a little pin on her obi (a fabric belt that is a distinctive part of the Jedi costume). The pin was a TARDIS. The "Mara" Jedi was not Mara Jade at all, she was Amy Pond (the Doctor Who companion, who I had also completely identified with and had begun to cosplay constantly) as a Jedi!

I made a new friend, a friend who was actually a fellow Amy and Leia cosplayer. And that is where the slippery slope began. I try not to be jealous of other cosplayers or how many events they get to attend per year, but Kristin, my Ginger Jedi, was living the dream as a Leia in the Rebel Legion. She had the dress, hair, boots - everything - along with Stormtroopers for miles. And she was attending event after event. I convinced myself I could never be that good, and that I would never want to interfere with all the fun she was having. She kept encouraging me to do Leia. I would explain that I had and that I even still had the dress in storage but that wasn't my life anymore. And in storage the dress stayed, for a while, until I got word that Kristin was leaving NYC and moving to the Washington D.C. area.

She told me it was my time, "I pass the buns to you. New York City needs a Princess!" So, I decided to give it a try. I still had the dress after all, now almost twenty years old, stained, and living in a storage box. To my surprise the stains came out. I made a new belt, ordered boots, and went to my first event. Even though I still wasn't a member of the Rebel Legion, and I was unclear how all of that worked, I was back in the outfit of the Princess. That first event back in the buns for me was the Star Wars Night at Citi Field, during a New York Mets baseball game. I don't remember the game, but I was to blown away by the reaction I received from the crowd. I shouldn't say 'I' because it wasn't me...it was Leia. So many people, young, young at heart, big guys and little girls, all came up to tell me how much Leia meant to them. Hands waving from afar, shy faces peering around parents just to get a look.

I had thought I was the only one... I was wrong.

I cannot express the power that is Leia. There has always been a special connection to the character. But then The Force Awakens was released, and the Princess was now a General. The effect of those few scenes from this new movie of a much older Leia (but one with the same feisty spark and command over all the boys) was profound, and this new movie would carry on that connection to a new generation too. The new character of Rey would do the same for 5 year old girls now as Leia had done for me, but with the General now there to guide it all. I didn't think we could love her more, but we did.

2016 was the year I decided I would finally meet Carrie Fisher. I had blown my chance 3 years earlier at New York Comic Con, thinking I shouldn't spend the money. I was an idiot. But now was my chance; I just had to find a convention where she was appearing. But as I looked for the right chance, I had to plan out what I was going to say. "Hi Ms. Fisher, I have been a fan of yours since I was 5 years old!" Great, that's what every fifty something wants to hear from someone who is obviously not a kid anymore. Did I want to bring up the looks thing? What would happen if I did and she just looked at me and said, "I don't see it?" I didn't know what to do. Then I started thinking about the "compliments" that I had gotten most of my life. It went like this, "Hey do you know who you look like? No not now when she is old and fat, the young hot version!" The rudeness of people can be dumbfounding. It happened so often that I got to the point where I knew where it was going and I would cut them off, "I understand what you are trying to say, and thank you, she is very beautiful even today." Most people would take the hint and back off.

Of course, this same issue was sometimes brought up to Carrie Fisher herself and she would use one of the sharpest minds and greatest wits ever put on earth to show us all how to deal with an idiot. "Please stop debating about whether or not I have aged well. Unfortunately it hurts all three of my feelings. My BODY hasn't aged as well as I have. Blow us!" This was a woman who was still shaping who I was and I was proud. And with those responses, I had found what I wanted to say when I met her: "It takes an incredible person to inspire both a 5 year old and 45 year old in the same way. Thank you for being my light."

It turned out that the 2016 New York Comic Con would be my chance. I got my ticket for the photo and I had my time to line up in the giant queue. Then, I just had to actually make it through the wait. At least as I waited, I had two of the greatest people in my life trying to keep me from passing out. As we stood in the queue tons of Leias walked past, and a funny realization dawned on me. I knew almost every one of them, hundreds of people. All Leias. Either in person or online, I knew most of these ladies, my Bun Sisters.

Finally it was my time, I was next in line. I was shaking so hard with so many emotions, holding the hands of my friends to try to stay grounded as I practiced what I had decided to say to her. But then she turned, and she smiled… You know that look your Mom or Grandma can give you when you do something so greatly unimportant or unimpressive and they just beam at you as if you are the greatest thing in the world? As I stood there in my white dress and my space buns, that is the look that was on Carrie's face and she reached out both her hands to me and said, "Look at you." I was done.

I held her hands and tried to talk but no words came. For 6 months I've been practicing and all I could squeak out was "I love you, thank you." She answered back, "I love you too." I got a hug and a pic and as I stumbled out I also got a "woof" from a very sleepy Gary (Gary Fisher, Carrie's support dog who would accompany her everywhere, including to convention and event signings). I patted his adorable head and literally bounced out of the photo area.

As I spoke to my friends after that, it became obvious both actress and character had touched so many of us. My friend Amy, who was adopted, was amazed as a small child to discover on a package of a doll the following words, "Princess Leia, adopted daughter of Bail Organa of the Royal house of Alderaan." A Princess? Adopted? This wound up meaning the world to little Amy. This was Leia. Important, connecting, loving. Another friend, Kelly, after getting her photo signed, thanked Carrie for showing her that she didn't have to choose between being a writer and an actress. Carrie then reached over, pulling the photo back and added under each of their names "WRITER/ACTRESS". This was Carrie. Genuine, real, loving.

But I had failed in my mission. I had wanted to tell her in words what she meant to me, and I had missed the chance. Luck, however, was on my side. Just a month later, Carrie began her book tour for *The Princess Diaries* and a bookstore in the city would hold a signing event. That night we stood in the cold, freezing our butts off, praying for a stray tauntaun to wander through lower Manhattan. When I got to her, we chatted about the purple streak in her hair and that I got a chance to meet her at NYCC but while I was there the words wouldn't come out. I was once again meeting this amazing writer and actress – a master of words – and I felt like a sputtering idiot. As I laughed, she looked at me and I burbled, "This is so crazy, every time I try to tell you how you have impacted my life, the words don't come out. Thank you for being you. Thank you for being so damn awesome!" She smiled and reached across the counter, taking my hand and looking into my eyes in a way that I could feel it in the back of my head. "I hear you, the words are there. They are leaving your mouth and touching my heart." I cry-laughed and through my sniffling said, "Don't ever stop being a badass." She chuckled, saying she had no intention to.

Then December arrived.

My sweetheart Clay and I had traveled to Georgia so I could meet his family and celebrate the holidays with them. We had plans for a night of bowling and arcades with the kids; I had a slight headache and I laid down that afternoon to get rid of it before our night out. I woke up from my nap around 3 PM, picked up my phone and opened Facebook to see "Carrie Fisher suffers in-flight heart attack, without oxygen for 15 minutes." The news hurt, it hurt a lot. But if anyone could pull through it would be my Princess – she was the poster child of a fighter. I tried to have fun that night, I really did. Friends and family reached out to me to see if I was okay, and an overwhelming flow of support and love began coming my way, as if I could pass it along to her and let her know we were thinking about her.

Then it happened.

Days had passed, and there had been no good announcements. I spoke to my friends and I steeled myself. I was mostly just glad that I was alone in the office at the time that the final news that she had died came in. I just put my head down.

As soon as we lost Carrie my social media exploded, hundreds of messages of love and loss flooded my page, private messages, texts, and phone calls. Even my gruff and businesslike boss came in, expressing his surprise that I was still at work. He had been in a Broadway Bowling league with Carrie and her mom, the great Debbie Reynolds (who sadly passed away the day after her beloved daughter). The news was affecting everyone. And everyone wanted to share their loss with me.

It became overwhelming. But in the midst of it all, I realized, this was a way for others to reach out and make a connection with someone they knew would understand their grief. People had created a virtual wake, and I, with my homemade costume and my doe eyes, had become one of the hosts. I was in charge of the guest book. I decided at that point that I had to do something to carry on. I had to do this for Carrie.

When January finally came and it was time to show the worst year of our lives out the door, I decided to kick it off by finally conquering my oldest fear, needles. I went in and I got a tattoo for Carrie, a tiny Rebel Bird on my wrist. The whole time I was there her words ran through my head, "Be afraid, but do it anyway." I felt like such a badass.

When the time came for me to attend my first convention since losing our princess, I started to worry. I had been planning to bring mostly Leia costumes and enter my Ceremonial dress in the Masquerade. But after all that had happened, was it too soon? Not just for me but for the other attendees? The deciding factor was the children's hospital visit I had scheduled soon after. I needed to rip off this Band-Aid now, and not risk getting teary eyed around little ones who needed me to be strong. The Princess had to be ready, but I didn't know if I was.

I know this sounds dramatic, but it weighed heavily on my mind. I was still receiving messages, texts, and posts on my Facebook wall memorializing Carrie. She was at the forefront of so many people's minds. I finished putting on the dress, makeup, and setting the hair and stepped out the door. As I made my way to the elevators, that's when I heard an audible gasp.

I turned. A woman in a beautiful Italian renaissance gown had stopped in her tracks feet away from me. She shook her head and tried to apologize but as I looked up from the floor, where I had buried my eyes in the hopes of hiding, it didn't stop her reaction, the old words, but they sounded different, "You look just like her." She just stood there for a second. Then she reached out to me, touching my arm. "Thank you for this, it's like she is still here." I can't think of anything I would have been less prepared for. She said, "Can I give you a hug?" I thanked her and gave her the hug, expressing how we all missed Carrie. There were tears in her eyes.

We parted, but the sensation didn't leave me. My head was telling me, "go back to the room, and hide under the bed" but what my heart said was, "I can be there. Be at the con and remind others that Carrie was still there in our hearts." And so that is what I did. I took my first steps into a much larger world.

The day was filled with photographs, and people's stories, the bonding of hearts in grief, everyone missed her and I knew they did. There was an endless stream of "You know who you look like? I bet you get that all the time." But my new heartfelt response was, "Yes!", because now I cannot hear it enough.

Of course, there were also new difficulties. There was the young man with his caregiver that kept following me around and pointing to my face shouting, "GHOST!" After about the fourth time I finally got it. I figured out it was the only way he could put into words what he was feeling, but it still chilled me to the bone. Then there was the muggle, the non con goer, who came up to me as we were leaving dinner. A group of ladies smiled and told me I looked great. I thanked them with a smile. The love that people were expressing for her was so powerful. Then the jerk who was with them opened his mouth, "Aren't you dead?" No retaliation or amount of words would stop the sickening feeling in my stomach. I just walked away. This man didn't know me, he couldn't possibly understand or comprehend what pain I felt. But my heart broke as the reality broke over me. There are some people who take pleasure in others' pain and laugh at loss. The world really does have a long way to go.

Now six months have passed and the pain is still there, knowledge of how Carrie left us burned through the internet, changing nothing in the hearts of the people who love her. I have attended at least twenty events in the months since Carrie left us. The looks and the stares and the smiles have not ceased.

Today, as I travel home from a convention on the NYC Subway, a young lady in her twenties dressed in a very nice Harley Quinn costume approached me with a look of surprise on her face and she pressed her hands to her cheeks. She walked toward me and in a shaking voice said, "I never got to meet her! I miss her so much." Tears welled in her eyes and all I could do is ask if I can give her a hug. She said yes.

This is my blessing, my role in this world right now. Grief is a funny thing, and 2016 took so many great people away from us. Rickman, Bowie, Prince, Baker (our beloved R2-D2), and all of them are missed so much. But it was Carrie who made that initial connection with that 5 year old staring at the stars. After Carrie's passing I had a choice. I could cut people off and tell them my grief was personal. I could thank them but tell them that I was not able to deal with their grief on top of my own. I could smile, take the compliment, and walk away.

But those choices would not be Carrie's choice. She was notoriously giving! There are so many stories of her leaving an autograph session only to return with gifts for people in line. Or taking random people into her home. Or just sitting and listening to people's stories. That is the person I want to be. I want to not just the have face of the Princess, but also to have the heart. I want to be that light, to be just a spark of the glorious glow that was Carrie. We all need to keep that light in this world.

So I listen, I cherish their stories, their looks, and even the billions of times I hear, "Do you know who you look like?" I can't hear it enough now! All of that means that she is still alive and well in the hearts and minds of people. When they see her in me it means that she is in them and part of who they are. This happens everywhere, at Cons, in stores, on the subway, at my apartment building. One day, as I got off an elevator I heard two beautiful French ladies I had never seen before whisper to each other, "Oh mon dieu, elle ressemble à Carrie Fisher."

This is my job now, to keep her light alive and to remind people who she was, what she did, what she stood for. I want to keep reminding people that she loved us just as much as we loved her. And she would also want us to push and love and change the world around us for the better too.

While I have shed tears, gotten choked up, the ugly cry is still locked away, deep inside of me, like Leia's tears for Alderaan. When it finally comes, and it certainly will, I predict it will be at the entrance of a certain badass General in The Last Jedi. I find it ironic that this is the one emotion that I can compartmentalize and trap away. I am not excited for the movie to come. I want it always to be on the horizon, a constant promise of more Leia, of more Carrie.

Star Wars

So carry on and "Carrie on" in all that you do. Live life with a "no fucks given" abandon that would make our Princess proud of us. Take all this world has to offer, be a light to others, and leave this galaxy and all the creatures you meet better for having your light shine on them.

"Carrie on!"

HITCHHIKER'S GUIDE TO THE GALAXY
"Driven by Infinite Improbability"
by Andy Hicks

Far out in the uncharted backwaters of the unfashionable end of the Western Metro suburbs of Boston lies a small, unregarded little town. One of the former residents of this town was an utterly insignificant little pale-skinned nerd, who, as our story opens, was so amazingly primitive that he still thought Hypercolor t-shirts and fanny packs were a pretty neat idea.

This child has – or, rather, had – a problem, which was this: most of the people he knew seemed to be setting up weird and arbitrary systems that didn't make any sense and only served to complicate matters. He'd spent the last few years at an elementary school designed around the "open classroom" theory. The idea was, a town would build a very large classroom. They would then section that classroom off into five segments: four "class areas", and one big meeting place in the middle. Having done all that, the final step would be to drop roughly 120 screaming children, and four teachers, into the large, arena-like space, shut the doors, close the windows, turn up the radiator, and sit back, confident in the knowledge that you've revolutionized public education by eliminating outdated, nonsensical concepts like "a controlled environment" and "learning."

It was 1990. The earthling's name was Andy Hicks. He was a ten-year old ape descendant with undiagnosed predominantly inattentive attention deficit disorder (ADHD/PI) and co-morbid rejection sensitive dysphoria, and a book is about to drive a bypass through his soul.

This is not his story.

Hitchhiker's Guide To The Galaxy

I mean, it kind of is. But mostly, it's the story of *The Hitchhiker's Guide To The Galaxy.*

If *Hitchhikers' Guide* feels like something that was made up as the author went along, that's because it was. The thing is, it works.

The first reason it works is that the disjointed nature of the narrative underscores the main theme of the books, which is – essentially – the story of man's search for meaning in a universe where petty bureaucracies, bloody-minded machine-logic, and decisions made with no thought about how those decisions might affect others, aren't just human failings, they're *universal* failings. The local government decided that Arthur Dent's house would be knocked down to build a bypass, and failed to properly communicate that fact with him, or anyone else. Then the Vogons show up, and blow up the Earth *for the exact same reason.* The story is so familiar by this point that we kind of forget how brilliant that is.

The second reason is because "making things up as he went along," was pretty much Douglas Adams's superpower. See, the first episode of the *Hitchhiker's Guide* radio show was actually supposed to be the first episode of an anthology series called *The Ends Of The Earth.* Next week, you were supposed to hear a completely different take on how the planet could conceivably blow up, and so on.

But then, Douglas remembered being 19 years old, lying drunk in a field while hitchhiking through Europe. He'd been reading a book called *The Hitchhiker's Guide To Europe,* and – as he stared up at the night sky – thought it would be cool if someone wrote a similar book about the whole galaxy. Having decided that his alien-invasion-via-incompetent-bureaucracy story needed a character who knew what was going to happen before anyone else, he then thought "hey, this guy – let's call him Ford Prefect - should be a field researcher for... *The Hitchhiker's Guide To The Galaxy*!"

(For maximum effect, please read those last two paragraphs while listening to "Journey Of The Sorcerer" by The Eagles.)

The whole story is held together by Adams' extremely strong comedic point of view, which keeps us tethered even as he gleefully bounces from idea to idea. The Earth is demolished. Vogons torture you by forcing you to listen to awful poetry. Our heroes then get rescued by a spaceship that's, appropriately enough, powered entirely by randomness. There's a mythical world that – as legend tells it – got extremely rich by building planets. And – oh, wait for it – it turns out that the Earth was, in fact, a giant supercomputer! See, millions of years ago, a couple of philosophers had wanted to know the true meaning of life, the universe, and everything, and they built a big computer called Deep Thought to crunch the numbers, and the answer it finally spit out, after millions of years of calculating was – all together now – 42.

Once the computer delivered that answer though, it also announced that the problem was they hadn't actually agreed on what the *question* was, so they decided to design another computer to figure that one out, and – lo and behold – it was the Earth. And then, mere hours before the Earth would have figured out what the *question* was, the Vogons went and blew it up.

It's the only time - in the original story, at least – where there's any kind of obvious setup and payoff, but it's a big one. The reason nothing makes sense on Earth, is because Earth was created specifically so that someone else could figure out why nothing made sense anywhere else. You could read this to mean that the world we live on – the rules we make for ourselves, the ways we communicate, and the ways we fail to communicate – are a distilled microcosm of the ineffably chaotic nature of the universe itself.

Anyway, back to Fifth grade.

Zoom in on weird little Andy, doing long division and utterly failing to carry the two and winding up with a remainder that's way more complicated than it should be. Cut to: his teacher, joking in front of the class that his "answers were on steroids," which was funny the first two or three times, maybe. Cut to: the other kids in class, picking up on the fact that "even the teacher makes fun of Andy," and – despite the fact that, last week, they were picking on him for being too smart – are now picking on him because his *math* is weird.

In fact, there are a lot of things about Andy that are "weird." He drops *Star Trek* references in class, and *Star Trek* is weird. He sings pop songs in the hallway on his way to the bathroom. He's hyperactive and gets into trouble because he isn't careful, but he's also kind of a goody-goody and doesn't like being rough and violent like boys are supposed to be. He reads. For fun. His parents don't even have cable. They lead the music at church, and some of the kids go to the same church and they see his parents up there leading music at church, and that's weird. And what's really weird, is that sometimes, when they make fun of him for all the little weird things he does like talking about *Star Trek* and singing and just being weird, he gets really mad and spazzes out on whoever's nearby. Like, at random.

Andy – for his part - doesn't know why he has to go to this school, and why it's somehow his fault for "bringing it on himself" instead of their fault for punching him and tripping him and calling him names. If there are rules governing this world, he doesn't know what they are. They seem really arbitrary. For instance, back in second grade, some other kids hog-tied him and his best friend to each other at recess. Supposedly, it was all part of a game. Then the bell rang, and everyone ran in, leaving them there. When they finally got untied, they ran straight to the main office... and got in trouble for coming in from recess late.

The Hitchhiker's Guide To The Galaxy is – allegedly - way too advanced for a ten year old. And yet, for me, it made all the sense in the world.

Douglas Adams was tall. Really, really tall. You won't believe just how mind-bogglingly tall Douglas Adams was. He was so tall, in fact, that on school trips, when most teachers would say "meet under the fountain" or "meet under that tree," his teachers told their classes to "meet under Adams."

One day, he was playing rugby, and his ungainly awkward knee came in contact with his ungainly awkward nose, permanently damaging his cartilage and making it impossible for him to breathe through his nose for the rest of his life.

He missed deadlines. Possibly his most famous quote that isn't actually in one of his books is "I love deadlines. I love the whooshing noise they make as they go by." He constantly delivered books late, or had to be locked in hotel rooms with his computer until they were finished. In fact, the reason that the first *Hitchhiker's* book only adapted the first four episodes of the original six-episode radio series, was that the book had been delayed so long that the publisher apparently just sent someone to Douglas' house to collect the manuscript in whatever form it was in. That's why it sort of just... ends, with a perfunctory one-page chapter where Zaphod Beeblebrox announces that they're heading to "the Restaurant at the End of the Universe."

And yet, people loved collaborating with the guy, regardless of how frustrating it was, because he was constantly churning out ideas. He saw connections between things that no one else saw. He thought about what might be possible with computers, and how they might affect publishing and the flow of information, and – voila – there's the titular Hitchhiker's Guide – a portable information terminal that connects to a vast network of articles, images, and sounds. In 1979, it must have seemed like an artifact from the distant future. In 2017, you have one in your pocket. He was a genius at figuring out how people might relate to technology, and also a genius at pinpointing the specific ways technology wasn't living up to its promise – whether he was directing his satirical rage at a Nutrimatic drink dispenser that couldn't figure out how to make tea, or at any personal computer not manufactured by Apple.

I'm not saying that Douglas Adams had ADHD/PI, because I'm not a medical professional and, even if I were, it is unbecoming to diagnose the dead. Having said that, he had all the symptoms. It takes one to know one.

The *Encyclopedia Galactica* has this to say on the subject of People With ADHD: "Attention Deficit Hyperactivity Disorder is a neurodevelopmental disorder that affects certain carbon based life forms, believed to be caused by functional impairments in the brain's neurotransmitter systems, particularly involving dopamine and norepinephrine receptors."

The Hitchhiker's Guide To The Galaxy also mentions ADHD. To paraphrase: Sometimes, we're Arthur Dent, and the world doesn't make a damn bit of sense, we can't ever seem to get a foothold, the rules keep changing, and we're still in our pajamas. Everyone thinks we're dumb and useless, and we can stumble into manipulative situations without realizing it. At our best, though, we're persistent. We ask the questions no one else is asking, even if people think we're dumb. "Is there any tea on this spaceship?" Or "Why can't we use the infinite improbability drive to destroy the missiles?"

Or, if we're talking specifically about Douglas Adams... well, dust off that old copy of *The Salmon Of Doubt* and flip to the essays he wrote for MacUser and The Independent in the '80s and '90s, and you'll see him asking things like "why can't we access high speed internet on mobile devices?" and "so, why can't I start a document on my desktop computer, and then have it instantly show up on my laptop?" That last one was from 1989. The guy predicted Google Docs in 1989. He wasn't a soothsayer or a wizard – he was just a guy who'd lost a few good chapters when the electricity went out, and frequently forgot to save his work. They say necessity is the mother of invention, but sometimes necessity is the unholy love child of failure and distraction.

Every now and then, we're Zaphod Beeblebrox, but only when we've somehow divorced ourselves of our self-awareness. Most of the time we hate people like Zaphod because nothing bothers us more than someone who's dumb, happy, and cocky. Here we are, trying really, really hard **not** to be dumb – pushing ourselves to perfection, second guessing everything we do – and meanwhile this guy swoops in, turns towards the attractive person we're flirting with, and says "Hey, doll, why don't you come and talk to me? I'm from a different planet." I mean, seriously. The guy gets away with stealing a spaceship and I can't even do long division properly.

Hitchhiker's Guide To The Galaxy

Sometimes we're Trillian, who got so bored with the dreary life of academia that she ran off with a two-headed alien she met at a party. Folks like us tend to make hasty decisions, crave novelty, and sometimes wind up in unhealthy situations as a result – no matter how "devastatingly intelligent" we are. Her characterization in Adams' final Hitchhikers book, *Mostly Harmless*, is even more poignant: that's where we meet an alternate universe version of Trillian who *didn't* leave with Zaphod, and who became a TV news reporter instead. She's still got the double degrees in math and astrophysics, though, and parallel universe/"what if?" themes crop up throughout.

I could write a whole separate essay about how this manifests itself in the various "official versions" of *Hitchhiker's Guide*, and how they all diverge from each other and contradict themselves so heavily that there's no such thing as a proper continuity. Suffice it to say, Douglas Adams never let "established canon" get in the way of pushing his characters into radically new situations every time the story hopped from one medium to another. He built himself a world where he could always go back and take a different path.

And sometimes, at our worst, we're Marvin the Paranoid Android. Because we're taking in so much information, all the time, and don't have the ability to process it all, we focus on what feels important. And, sometimes, the sense of self-protection we've built for ourselves against the onslaught of data totally backfires, and the only thoughts and feelings we can process are the negative ones. Psychiatrists call this "rejection sensitive dysphoria." Because we're never quite sure when we're letting people down until it's too late – and we're *always* letting people down, it seems – folks with ADHD occasionally have a tendency to over-correct, and just assume that everyone wants us to go stick our heads in a bucket of water.

Sometimes, however, we're Ford Prefect. And these are the times when we're in our element, we've sussed out the situation, we know where the good parties are, and we really know where our towel is. See, an ADHD/PI-type spends most of their life alternating between a dreamy, lazy state, and a panicked, "where the hell are my keys?" state. And while this is not a particularly tenable position to constantly find oneself in, one does manage to exercise both the "creative problem-solving" and "dealing with crisis" parts of one's brain quite often. That means, if there's something you happen to be good at, you're *really* good at it. If there's a particular social setting you feel comfortable in, you'll make a lot of friends and be really, really cool.

You might be an alien, but your perspective doesn't necessarily *alienate* you. You might notice things no one else notices. You might be able to slide effortlessly into any number of settings, and go off on great adventures, and know about all the neat stuff the normal people *don't* know about. If you can disguise yourself as "one of them" for just long enough to get by, you'll do all right. Heck, you'll do better than all right. Because – at the end of the day, at the end of the *universe* even - it's all about knowing where your towel is.

March 8, 1978. *The Hitchhiker's Guide To The Galaxy* premieres on BBC 2. Almost no one listened to that first episode, apparently. The show became a hit through word of mouth. And one of the things that really struck people, once they actually heard it, was how different it sounded. See, radio drama never really died in England, though most radio comedies back then still sounded like they had thirty years previous. You know: live studio audience, live Foley effects with coconuts clopping for horses, and so on. *Hitchhiker's*

— on the other hand — was produced more like a rock album. There's explosions, computer blips, synthesized ambient hums, ring modulated alien voices, wisps of atmospheric music... all kinds of things radio drama listeners are used to hearing *now*, but — believe you me — *Hitchhiker's* did it first. It's classic fish-out-of-water comedy by way of Pink Floyd. It's an idea that's simultaneously out-of-left-field, and yet completely obvious once you think about it.

One of our local Boston stations happened to air it in the winter of 1991. I was eleven years old. I can still remember sitting in the front seat of my father's old van, driving through a winter storm, while the opening music plunked away under Peter Jones' comforting narration. The way the headlights illuminated the snowflakes in the darkness as we drove onwards through the night, I swore I was flying through hyperspace.

And in a way, I was — escaping from the mean kids at school, the forgotten homework assignments that seemed to mean so much at the time, the fear that I'd never belong. Traveling light years ahead, into a future full of darkness and light. I was a year away from my first starring role in a play, and two years away from my first serious depressive episode. In four, I'd start writing my own songs. Five years, my first sound design. Six years, I'd make the wrong college choice on a whim and feel completely alienated — and then, eventually, completely *accepted*, all over again, and I wouldn't quite understand any of it.

Ten years and four months later, I'd be writing a parody of the opening song for "Cabaret" for our college theater departments' end of year roast and awards banquet, in my girlfriend's dorm room, when I'd learn that

Douglas Adams – the author who told me, whether he realized it or not, that it was okay to be weird - had died suddenly at a gym in California.

It's a genuine tragedy that the guy who predicted the iPhone didn't even live long enough to own an iPod. Sometimes, the Vogons blow up your planet before you even know what the question is.

In twelve years, I'd get my first professional job in radio. In nineteen years, I'd be working for a different station – the very same station, in fact, where I had heard the first episode of *The Hitchhiker's Guide To The Galaxy* on that starry, snowy night in 1991. There will be long periods of confusion, anger, elation, uncertainty, and the inability to get a nice cup of really hot tea. I will run off with people who claim to be from a different planet.

The world will end, several times.

And I'm still here.

And – every now and then – I almost feel like I know where my towel is.

HARRY POTTER
"Breaking the House Rule"
by Clay Dockery

"Which House are you?"

At just about any gathering of Harry Potter fans this is the very first, and most fundamental question. The answer you give will create your community and also set boundaries that may last for years. House identity to Potter fans is both fully subjective and almost absolutely amorphous. The houses become your pack, your biggest supporters and your bulwark to the world. And because of that, I have become most fascinated with studying the phenomena, with attempting to understand how and why people are drawn to a specific house identity and what it is about the identities that compels people to each. But how did we get here, what makes this question so important and essential to Harry Potter fans, and why is it almost always the first thing any Potter fan is asked?

When the Harry Potter series was first published, I was not particularly into children's books, or stories about wizards, or even the fantasy genre as a whole. I was known (and still am in some circles) as a cantankerous and demanding person who found it difficult to truly get fully invested in new things. It took a very long time for people to convince me to read the three (at the time) books about a boy wizard. It took even longer for me to agree to participate in discussions with the fandoms. It was much longer still before I agreed to meet people involved in the fandom in person. Now, seventeen years later, these people, those books, this story has shaped my entire life in ways I would have never thought possible.

After nearly a year of saying, "that story isn't for me" and avoiding any mention of the stories, I finally decided to read *Harry Potter and The Sorcerer's Stone* just before the first movie was released in November of 2001. It was still far from something I was enthusiastic about doing. My thought process was basically to get the book out of the way because I figured someone would eventually either want to go to the movie with me, or it would come on TV and I would then be forever in a world where I saw the movie first, and even though I had no real interest in the story, I definitely didn't want that.

As I read the story I distinctly remember the stages I went through in my head: First chapter- "this flashback is silly, but the little details are pretty funny." Second chapter- "ugh, it is one of those stories where the orphan is raised by horrible people." and so on. There were definitely high points and interesting parts, but the first six chapters even with Hagrid and the owls, Diagon Alley, and the Hogwarts Express didn't really grab me. And then I hit chapter six, "The Sorting Hat" and as the door to Hogwarts swung open to reveal a tall witch in emerald green robes, the story began to take me on a journey that will last for the rest of my life.

As that witch, Minerva McGonagall, introduced the rules and structures of the school I was transfixed, not just because a tall stern woman in command will always get my attention, but also because of the specific words Rowling used to describe these "Houses". "The four Houses are called Gryffindor, Hufflepuff, Ravenclaw, and Slytherin. Each House has its own noble history and each has produced outstanding witches and wizards... I hope each of you will be a credit to whichever House becomes yours." And with that introduction the story truly began to take shape and would etch itself into my mind. This was not just a story of an outsider kid, or even a hero's journey (while of course it is also those things); this story establishes right there that it is about identity. What it takes to be a part of a group, why we associate with the people we do, and how our goals and aspirations are influenced by our circumstances and associations, as much as our talents.

As I continued to read, I kept getting drawn back to those themes time and again. *Sorcerer's Stone* is a very short book and before I really realized it, I had finished reading it never all that interested in the plot, but compelled by the character's search for meaning and belonging. I had purchased a package with the first three books and before the night was over I had read all three. The Prisoner of Azkaban sealed my interest in the story itself as well as introducing the character that I personally identify with the most, Remus Lupin, but my connection to the story had already become profound and unbreakable by that point.

Before I continue the story of my own journey, let's take an aside into the notion of connection and think for a moment about the meaning of these relationships. What is it that made this connection to the story possible? The plots and characters of the stories are interesting but, especially in those early books, not particularly exceptional or enlightening. The structure of the world and mixture of humor and pathos are both intriguing aspects but are aspects of hundreds of other stories that don't have the same level of connection and commitment from readers. In his well-regarded books on classical theory and religion in the Harry Potter series, John Granger (known as "The Hogwarts Professor") has argued that Joanne Rowling tapped intentionally into a set of Classical and deeply Jungian mysteries. Yet, despite the compelling nature of his work (his "Ring Cycle" theories in particular are quite exceptional) I do not believe that is the case.

While there are definitely archetypical "hero's journey" aspects to the stories, I have never fully bought into the idea that they are somehow cosmically transcendent. I think that the connection I feel and the main connection that most permeates the entire fandom that has developed around these stories is to the very real and explicit invitation the book makes for us to build an identity for ourselves. Our identities are developed within the "Wizarding World" and then we can use those tools to express that identity back into our everyday lives.

The most basic form of that connection hinges on the concept of house identity. People have been creating groupings and various labels to try to express identity for thousands of years. In most cases there is a proscription to the label: it is something given by others and one either attempts to reconcile that label with who they are, or they are forced to abandon it entirely. Or the label is about something you do or like, but not an attempt to fundamentally express who you are. Most of our experiences with fandoms fall into this category. I might be a hard core follower of the Galactic Solar Olympics or a drinker of the effervescent Doctor Juniper Juice but the other followers may all be Minotaurs from the Mines of Moria and we have nothing in common at all. House identity, and with it fundamentally Harry Potter fandom itself, is not that way at all. House identity is both a shared communal experience, determined by everyone and also a deeply personal, fundamentally existential decision.

In the story, the sorting hat chooses which house each student should be placed within, but the hat does not do it arbitrarily, or even alone. The sorting is based primarily on the skills and talents of the sortee but also with an element of what the sortee wishes their skills and talents might be. Within this world the identity of the person is not deterministic; while there are aspects of all identity that are necessarily so, neither our own skills and talents nor the identity that has been given to us by others fully contains who we really are.

So, while each house is given a set of traits and characteristics that sets it apart from the others, the actual decision to become a member of that house is most set by the idea of what the sortee desires. The traits are aspirational, the houses calling each student to see those things that they value most and then allowing them to choose to follow that path in their schooling, and due to the way the universe is structured, therefore in their lives. By allowing for this choice to be determined in this way, Rowling has created a universe in which the divisions should be undercut from the very beginning. The fact that this idea is undercut in the story itself due to plot needs and an oversimplified rendering of one of the houses does not make it any less essential to the real people who have encountered the world. To connect these ideas it is important to compare how each of the houses are described by Joanne Rowling in the story to how most people who identify with the house see themselves.

In *Harry Potter and the Sorcerer's Stone*, Rowling has the "Sorting Hat" sing a song that forms the basis for the identity of the houses which will be expanded and deepened in the series, but the basic and essential elements remain the same throughout:

You might belong in Gryffindor,

Where dwell the brave at heart,

Their daring, nerve, and chivalry

Set Gryffindors apart;

You might belong in Hufflepuff,

Where they are just and loyal,

Those patient Hufflepuffs are true

And unafraid of toil;

Or yet in wise old Ravenclaw,

If you've a ready mind,

Where those of wit and learning,

Will always find their kind;

Or perhaps in Slytherin,

You'll make your real friends,

Those cunning folk use any means

To achieve their ends.

Gryffindor is the house that is most fully explored in the story. By virtue of being the house of the main characters there is more time to develop both their personalities and the ways in which those personalities tie them to their house. As such, it is easy to see the ways the traits fit the definition of the "hero's house." These traits reflect the needs of the protagonists of the story being told. Yet there is both a compelling aspect to the traits as presented, and an easy to uncover darkness. Gryffindors are brave, yes, but that bravery can lead to recklessness. Even in the most essential house for the narrative, the structure allows for layers: the identities of Ron, Harry and Hermione (and Neville) will be fully formed in time, but even from this first moment these indelible ideas deepen the characters.

Hufflepuff is another matter entirely. The traits of this house are not as well defined and are often used, both in the narrative and in fandom, in an effort to dismiss the house as "lesser than" the others, especially when the "Hufflepuff will take the rest" ideas from the Sorting Hat's later song are also included. But once again, in the lines themselves, and in the estimation of those people who identify with the house, there is a beautiful set of compelling traits that set Hufflepuffs apart, with the most essential being loyalty and dedication to friends. Hufflepuffs aren't "a bunch of duffers" toiling away at just anything: the toil they are engaged in is an attempt to actively build a world based on more compassionate values. This has become increasingly evident as more Hufflepuffs have been given prominent roles in Harry Potter stories, most essentially the fantastic Newt Scamander in the *Fantastic Beasts and Where to Find Them* film (which was also written by Rowling.)

The essential traits of Ravenclaw are relatively well established, but by virtue of having few major characters highlighted there can be a tendency to think of the connection to the house in a crude way. In most cases this leads to the simplistic "Ravenclaws are the smart House" line of thinking, along with the companion argument that "Hermione should have been in Ravenclaw." Neither of those lines of thought has ever been compelling to me; from these lines, and also from the most established Ravenclaw character, Luna Lovegood, it is clear that Ravenclaw is a house for those who are interested in the love of learning, the open mind, or the eccentric, more so than "being smart" or even valuing information.

Slytherin is easily the most complicated of the houses to parse, and is often the most easily misconstrued by everyone from characters within the story, to fans, to Rowling herself. The Slytherin characters, especially in the early stories, are presented as the villains, and there is already an inherent sense from many people that being overly ambitious is bad. In the fandom too, many people initially decided to "join the evil House" due to an affinity for villains or at least darkness. And by virtue of the fact that the house is associated quite readily with a racist, classist system imposed by its founder it is sometimes difficult for people to see beyond those aspects. (Including for Rowling herself, who once in an extremely misguided attempt to connect, told a young fan garbed in the green and silver, "Why would you ever want to be a Slytherin?")

And yet, those things are not the essential nature of the house as described in the story, and are not what most people find compelling about it. Instead, the house's connection for people is much more about creating and changing the world to allow for their unique self-expressions to grow and flourish. Ambition does not always lead to Tom Riddle's quest for immortality or a dictator's imposition of draconian systems, rather it can be about being able to be who you are, to actually express the fundamental self in a way that is accepted and valued. The story lets down the house in many ways, but it must be said that for all the faults the characters have, they are compelling and multi-layered. The Malfoy family lingers throughout the story on the edge, but draw you into the world as they see it by the end. And of course, with his complicated story and the deep flaws of the character,

Harry Potter

Severus Snape is perhaps the most compelling figure in the entire saga. All those aspects of those characters are deeply tied to their house, not as it relates to any sort of villainy, but as it relates to the constant tension between self-realization and self-actualization.

In all of the houses, though, there is a capacity for both good and bad, and there is a deeper connection to both classical theory of the humors and the four elements, as confirmed by Joanne Rowling herself on Pottermore.

> *The four Hogwarts houses have a loose association with the four elements, and their colours were chosen accordingly. Gryffindor (red and gold) is connected to fire; Slytherin (green and silver) to water; Hufflepuff (yellow and black, representing wheat and soil) to earth; and Ravenclaw (blue and bronze; sky and eagle feathers) to air.*
> - from "Colours" by J.K. Rowling at Pottermore.

All of the houses have something to offer the story, the characters, and the fandom. As the stories go on, the narrative deepens and the houses become much less strictly defined as the character's motivations are clarified. The story, and the fandom, have other great and interesting themes to explore. Yet it is usually through a house that fans become most attached to the tale, and it is so compelling that the fan's identity becomes forever intertwined with that house.

"And so, which House are you?" the proverbial questioner asks again. Instead of an answer, I continue my tale.

After reading the first three books, and becoming hooked on the universe, that first day I went back out and bought *Harry Potter and Goblet of Fire* and read it straight through without stopping as well. *Goblet of Fire* expanded upon and deepened everything that hooked me, and through the

53

establishment of the return of Voldemort and death of Cedric Diggory upped the stakes in a way that officially moved the entire series out of "children's literature I really like", to "literature I really like" in my mental categorization. And yet, while my own understanding of these stories was solidified I had not found the other people to discuss these ideas with, to grow and debate and argue and change each other. I had a few friends who also loved the story, but I had not yet found the fandom. I had no "House."

The early 2000s were an interesting time to be a burgeoning fan in any fandom, but in the Harry Potter fandom it was a truly transformative time. Joanne Rowling was actively writing the books, and as fans waited for the releases she would often make pronouncements about little details that would be gobbled up ravenously by everyone who heard them. Warner Brothers was making epic movies of those stories with an indelible cast of some of the greats of British theatre (and some pretty overmatched but charismatic teenagers as the leads.) Those twin behemoths catalyzed an amazing amount of creativity and connectivity among fans around the world, and with the internet also hitting its great peak of social connectivity and creativity the Harry Potter fandom exploded onto the world.

By late 2000 both MuggleNet and the Leaky Cauldron websites had been launched and both would serve as essential destinations for Potter fans from all over to get news about the series and films. Both would launch podcasts which became the voice of the fandom to most of the world. The Harry Potter sections of every great fan-fiction site filled to overflowing (including with full scale novel length alternative versions of books before their release). Fans flocked to LiveJournal and Yahoo message boards, "Harry Potter for Grownups" in particular, to discuss the series together. In 2002,

Harry Potter

two brothers (Paul and Joe DeGeorge) started a band called Harry and the Potters which would play music based on the series and would eventually spawn hundreds of bands and become its own genre, Wizard Rock (WROCK).

Nimbus 2003, the first Harry Potter "symposium", would usher in a series of increasingly large and diverse conventions specifically for the fandom. Around the country, meetup.com groups would form for monthly gatherings of fans, including TGTSNBN in New York City among many others. Harry Potter fandom had become something that could be a part of every aspect of life, but it wasn't yet that for me. I had not found my "House".

While I actually joined and participated very rarely during these early days of fandom beyond listening to PotterCast and having an account on the "Harry Potter for Grown Ups" listserv, it was still pervasive and formative. Throughout my time in graduate school I would read about the conventions and hear individual songs, of WROCK and think "hmmm, that sounds super cool, maybe someday I'll go to a convention." The community went on around me and intrigued me, but I was too busy and distracted by life to really hear the call.

As time passed by, I worked year after year at Summer Camp and shared each book release and movie premiere with small groups of friends and family my connection to the material deepened. I read each book immediately upon release and re-read the previous books once a year. I saw most of the movies the night they opened, even though I never liked them very much. I listened to the podcasts even as my participation on the forums waned. Finally, after *Harry Potter and the Deathly Hallows* (the seventh and final book) came out and the story was finished, I expected to drift entirely away from the story, and while I didn't think much about it, I expected the "fandom" would probably last through the rest of the movie releases and then drift away as well. I was entirely and profoundly wrong on both counts.

After working one final summer at camp in 2010, I changed the course of my life. I moved back to New York City, where I had gone to graduate school. Being alone in the city was difficult, I worked in an office with only two other people and had no other groups of friends still in the city. So, for the first few weeks I basically didn't speak to anyone in person outside of my office. Eventually, I decided I had to meet new people somehow and remembered that Meetup.com sometimes had interesting groups of people to join up with. I searched for hiking groups and book clubs, chat groups and bar hops. Nothing seemed remotely like it would work for me until I remembered two words and put them in the search bar: Harry Potter.

The Group That Shall Not Be Named, the NYC Harry Potter Meetup, was the first result. They met every month in the city and also had additional events and meetups at various times and places. There was a meetup that weekend and I decided to go. And then I freaked out, worried that I wouldn't fit in, or that the people would be too strange, or any number of other things. It would take me four tries and failures before I actually made it to my first event, a panel discussion on something I had never done, but which was super interesting to me: cosplay.

I went to the event, where a tall, scary, beautiful, redhead discussed the upcoming cosplay event, and I met the people, and it was a revelation. The subjects were interesting, the topics of the upcoming discussions compelling, and there was even a Harry Potter convention coming up in the following May. I was hooked. But I was also asked the question, probably 25 times since there were 25 people in the room, "What House are you in?" This time it was followed by the expectation of, "Who from that House would you cosplay?" I had borrowed my friend's Slytherin student robe and had affinity for Remus Lupin, so I said "Some from each?" and moved on. *I entered the cave.*

Since that first night, my life in the Harry Potter fandom has only grown. I not only attended the convention that next May, I have been the co-head organizer of three additional conventions and attended dozens of others. I started playing quidditch (yes there is substantial group of serious quidditch players in leagues around the world) and became involved in developing the rules, establishing even more long and essential friendships. (This has even led to different kind of "House Identity" with our annual "Ref Haus" shenanigans.)

After the final movies in the original series came out, the fandom did not fade – it shifted and changed and I moved with it. Harry Potter fandom has changed my life incredibly. It has led me to love and connection, renewal and rebirth, and allowed me to channel my creative energies into conventions and events and stories I never thought possible. In addition to the Potter fandom itself, it has been a gateway into every other fandom for me, where I participate as strongly— creating content and podcasts and conventions in those worlds too.

And through all of that, the most compelling aspects of the story remain wrapped up in the songs sung by that tattered old hat. I am drawn to discuss it, to dissect the reasons that we have these needs to self-identify and pair off, to berate the inadequacies of the Pottermore sorting tests and so on. To me, the story goes on forever and the self-identifying and sorting helps to make the story make more sense as we go along our journey.

"And so what House are you?"

I hold up my own ideals in the face of all the struggles of the world. I see the world, as I want it to be and though I may be flawed, I hope to help make it so. I am Lupin. I am a Gryffindor.

I hold the love of learning, of flying high into the stratosphere of my own delusions to be the most compelling life. I am Lovegood. I am a Ravenclaw.

I hold the love of friends to be sacred, that each relationship we make, that each creature we meet, needs to be tended to and cared for. I am Scamander. I am a Hufflepuff.

I hold the power to command and control the things that must be controlled to make things right. I know the ways and means to move ahead and accomplish what must be done, even if it is a struggle against my own self. I am Snape. I am a Slytherin.

So, what house am I anyway?

I am "House Curious", and I always will be.

BASEBALL
"Stitched Together"
by Betsy R. Shepherd

My obsession with baseball, particularly Atlanta Braves baseball, began at around 4 years old, when I first understood what baseball was and started watching the games on TBS with my dad. He had been a fan since the Braves moved to Atlanta in 1966. My dad is a quiet guy and it's not easy to really get to know him, but even as a preschooler I could see that Braves baseball was the key to doing just that. It was what he loved, so I learned to love it, too. My parents took me to my first Major League Baseball game in 1982 at the old Atlanta Fulton County Stadium. I loved riding the MARTA train downtown to go on this adventure. I loved the ballpark snacks. I loved being part of the cheering crowd. I loved everything about the team, despite the fact that they were terrible at playing baseball in those days.

Some of my earliest childhood memories are of sitting at the end of my parents' bed way past the time when I was supposed to be sleeping, begging to watch "just one more inning, Daddy," or "just until Dale Murphy bats again!" This tactic usually worked, but by the time I was 5 or 6 years old, it wasn't a ploy. I loved the game just as much as he did. I had a clock radio next to my bed and at night as I went to sleep I would listen to Pete Van Wieren and Skip Caray and Ernie Johnson describe the scene at the ballpark. It soothed my soul.

One spring day when I was 6, I went with my parents to the mall and they were having little league signups. There were tables for t-ball, baseball, and softball, and since I was a girl, my parents tried to steer me towards softball. I was insistent that "No, I'm going to play REAL baseball," so that was how I ended up being the sole female member of the Pinto League Tigers. My coach was a doctor in real life and turned out to be one of the nicest guys. He never made me feel like I was "less than", as some folks might have tried to do back then. I remember my dad teaching me to play catch in the backyard, how to grip the ball with two fingers instead of your whole hand, and how to put your whole body into the motion of throwing. I grew to love the smell of the leather glove and the wet, red Georgia clay lining the infield. I looked forward to every practice.

Being first graders, our games were only 5 innings long, but I remember wishing they were a full 9, and how thrilled I was the day we went into extra innings versus our biggest rivals, the Red Sox, and got to play 8. I would go to school and tell my teachers all about it. I know now that they were probably internally rolling their eyes at my post-game recaps of my Little League team, but at the time it seemed so very important to share every detail. I wasn't very good at Little League, although I gave it my all. Once the kids started pitching, the boys would deliberately throw at me for having the audacity to be a girl. My dad would have to stand by the fence the entire game just to make sure I was not being horribly mistreated. I remember one pitch hitting me square in the stomach and knocking the wind out of me, but instead of falling to the ground, I stood up and trotted to first base, much to the amazement of my coach, the umpire, the parents watching from the stands, and most especially the little 7-year-old creep who had thought his 20 mile per hour fastball was going to take me down.

On my ninth birthday, I had a party with all my friends at Stone Mountain Park. We climbed the mountain and then had a picnic of fried chicken and peanut butter sandwiches at the base of the rock. We knew Dale

Baseball

Murphy was at the mall that day signing autographs of his new book, *Ask Dale Murphy*, a series of advice column style questions and answers about baseball and his career. I had just gotten a copy of the book as a birthday gift. Because of the party, we weren't sure we were going to make it to the mall before Murphy had to leave for the game, but my dad drove like a bat out of hell and we somehow made it just in time. We were the last people they allowed in line before shutting the event down. I remember being mad that I was wearing a Hawaiian style shirt instead of my baseball jersey. When we got to the front of the line, I could hardly speak as my hero said hello and asked how I was doing. Grinning from ear to ear, "fine" was all I could manage to say. He couldn't have been nicer. It was a thrill like no other and the one childhood birthday I'll never forget.

Going to Braves games in person typically meant a great adventure with my dad. As I got a little older, the school system would give free pairs of tickets out to those of us who got good grades, so I ended up with lots of those. I was the oldest of four kids in my family, so one-on-one time with a parent was a coveted thing. We lived about a 20 minute drive from the stadium and I had all the neighborhoods along the way memorized from the backseat of my dad's Buick. My favorite view of the city of Atlanta skyline was from the south, as seen from the parking lot of the stadium. Dad always got us a program and we would study it together. He taught me how to keep score.

Sometimes I got to bring a friend on these adventures, and I chose which friend based on their ability to understand what was actually happening on the field without me having to explain and their ability to stay until the end of the game without getting fidgety and wanting to leave early.

There was nothing worse, in my nine-year-old estimation, than someone who saw the ballgame as an opportunity to gab about what was going on at school rather than as a near-holy event to be relished in exquisite detail the way I did.

My favorite friend to bring to ballgames was Andy. He lived down the street from us and was exactly 2 months older than me. We spent every day after school riding bikes, exploring the creek, trying to defeat Super Mario Brothers on our Nintendo, and playing endless games of backyard baseball with our brothers. All of those things were great, but our mutual love of baseball was what really drew me to Andy as one of my first real best friends. He didn't look at me like I was crazy when I talked about how I loved the smell of the dirt on the infield. He understood how to pause reverently when we walked into the stadium and glimpsed the grass for the first time. He paid attention to the game. On the ride home, we traded baseball cards in the backseat of my dad's car and I thought about how happy I was to have a friend like him who truly understood what was most important to me. He and his family moved away when I was 11 and although we tried to keep in touch for a while, the last time I spoke to him was on his 14th birthday. He was the same guy. He was happy I remembered his birthday, but for two kids who weren't old enough to drive and didn't have the benefit of the internet yet, the connection was too hard to keep up. I don't think I ever got over the heartbreak.

My dad's favorite place to park for Braves games was a hotel about 3 blocks away. It has changed names many times through the years, but at the time it was a Ramada Inn. We would stroll down the street, past the scalpers, through the pedestrian tunnel, and into the ballpark with the bag of peanuts my dad always had to grab on the way in. One night there were postgame fireworks, but we had my brother and one of his friends with us, and Dad had promised to have the friend home at a certain hour, so we had to duck out in the middle of the pyrotechnics. To get to the Ramada where we had parked, we had to cross through the restricted area where they were actually shooting off the fireworks. There were ropes and signs saying "road closed," but of course our dad said "it's not closed to ME" and ushered us all through to try to get to our car. Suddenly, flaming chunks of debris from the fireworks started landing all around us. We were running, but not fast enough. Dad happened to have an umbrella and he tried to use it to shield us from the shrapnel. Unbeknownst to him, my brother's friend stopped and picked up a piece of unexploded ordinance and showed it to him as we were about to get in the car. Trying not to freak out, Dad gingerly confiscated the item and set it down in the parking lot before we went on our way.

Dale Murphy was traded to the Philadelphia Phillies in August of 1990. I was 12 years old. It was a dark day in the city of Atlanta, and a darker day for me. I remember coming downstairs for breakfast and my dad had saved the sports page of the Atlanta Journal Constitution for me. I took it up to my room and laid on my bed and just stared at it in disbelief. I was about to start seventh grade, which was disconcerting enough, but seeing my hero move on to another city and another team was like the nail in the coffin of my childhood. I'm pretty sure no one in their right mind enjoys middle school, but that was a particularly rough year for me. I made a couple of important female friends, but they never did understand my baseball obsession, and how close can you really get to someone who doesn't have the key to your soul?

In the spring of 1991, the end of my seventh grade school year from hell, the Braves started to get really good. They had a new general manager, John Schuerholz, and he had traded for some great new players. My dad and I looked around the stadium during a night game in late April and noticed there were a lot more people than there had been in the past few years and we even spotted a vendor walking around selling souvenirs in the upper deck. I didn't recall having seen more than one concession stand open on the upper deck, let alone a souvenir vendor. That was our first clue that things were about to get really exciting. One night in May the Braves played the Pirates and the Braves' new first baseman, Sid Bream, who had just been traded to Atlanta from Pittsburgh, hit a grand slam against his old team. The crowd was so loud it was deafening. I had never experienced anything like that feeling in my entire life.

A couple of months later, my dad got a new job and we found out we were moving to Birmingham, Alabama. It was only two and half hours away, but for a 13-year-old, that is a life altering distance. I was devastated to be separated from my team just when they were having the best season I'd ever experienced. I even had to leave behind my local AM radio station where I listed to all the games to fall asleep at night. I spent an inordinate amount of time lamenting these losses. When we finally got to Alabama, I discovered we could at least continue watching the games on TBS, and sometimes late at night if I turned the radio dial just right, I could still pick up a faint signal from WSB. As fall approached, I picked up my old habit of sitting at the end of my parents' bed at the end of the evening watching "just one more inning" before I went to sleep. The Braves connection helped me make friends at my new school. It turned out there were other Braves fans in Alabama.

Baseball

One fall day in the band room, the drumline started a rendition of the tomahawk chant in the middle of class. The Braves were finally good again and everyone wanted to be in on the excitement. At home, my dad and I were beside ourselves when our team made the World Series. We stayed up way too late hanging on every pitch of all seven games. There was a TV downstairs in the living room, but for some reason we still gathered in my parents' bedroom around the tiny TV they had in there, with me and my brothers watching the games from sleeping bags on the floor. Kirby Puckett and the Minnesota Twins broke our hearts in the end, but that time of hope and possibility and family togetherness will be a light to me for the rest of my life.

The fall of 1995 was the beginning of my senior year of high school. In addition to being a Braves fan, I was very involved in my church and all of the youth activities that went along with it. School had never been much of a social outlet for me, and the only true friends I had in high school were through my church group. That was the reason I was torn between going on a community service retreat with those friends the weekend of Game 6 of the World Series or staying home to watch baseball. I ultimately decided that helping build houses for the poor was more important to me, but once I got out into the church camp setting in the woods, I just couldn't help myself. We happened to be having a camp-style communion service as the end of game six neared. I snuck someone else's Walkman out of the bunk house and surreptitiously tuned in from the back of the common room as the minister broke the bread and poured the wine. It seemed fitting that as that fly ball landed in Marquis Grissom's glove in center field for the final out and Skip Caray shouted "Yes! Yes!" I let out my own little whoop and scared the living hell out of all the kids seated around me. None of the adult youth leaders were pleased with me. All these years later, I'm still quite sure that God understands.

Baseball was never just a game to me, especially Braves baseball. It was my connection to my family, long lost friends, my entire childhood, and my understanding of my place in the world, and I think of those things as elements of my faith. I can't imagine a benevolent creator begrudging a person their moment of joy when a dream they've spent their whole life wishing for comes true. The only time my parents ever let me skip school was the following spring, to be present in Atlanta on Opening Day 1996 when the Braves' World Series rings were presented.

My college years were spent in Athens, GA, within an hour's drive of Atlanta. For the Olympics in 1996, the city built a new stadium, and after the games were over they converted it to a new baseball stadium for the Braves. When I went to my first game at the shiny new Turner Field, I sat in the upper deck, and I could see the old Fulton County Stadium still standing in darkness on the other side of the parking lot. It sounds silly now, but I felt like it was telling me it was okay to enjoy the new place and to move on. I still couldn't bring myself to watch the video of it being imploded later that year. Too many of my childhood memories happened in that spot. I grew to love Turner Field, though, and it had the same beautiful view of the downtown Atlanta skyline.

My sophomore year I met a young man, Clay, who shared my love of baseball and the Braves. One night we decided at the last minute to drive over to the stadium for the game and get some of the special one dollar nosebleed seats. I remember I only had $7 in cash to my name at the time.

Baseball

Luckily, that was enough for our tickets and one of those short cans of Pringles from the gas station as a snack for the road. I remember the feeling when we walked into the stadium together and glimpsed the grass for the first time and how astounded I was when he paused reverently with me and just appreciated that moment and the holiness of where we were. I think a part of me fell in love with him then.

I remembered Andy, my childhood best friend. Clay had just opened a little window into the part of myself I rarely shared with anyone else. That baseball connection is a powerful thing. As the years passed and things went to hell and back with the two of us romantically, Braves baseball became the one thing we could still talk to each other about without having a screaming fight. Eventually, we went our separate ways, but even from cities on opposite sides of the country I would still get the occasional message from him with a picture of a sunset from the upper deck of a ballpark somewhere.

After graduation I moved to New Mexico, far away from real baseball and my Braves. I learned how to snowboard and learned to love hiking in the Sangre de Cristo Mountains, and tried to fill that void with other things, but baseball never stopped tapping on my shoulder. I became a fan of Albuquerque's minor league team, the Isotopes. The team name came from an episode of the Simpsons. I grew frustrated with my law school friends, who were more interested in drinking beer and socializing than watching the games. I dated a series of guys and one of them, a physicist who worked at the Los Alamos National Laboratory, was smart enough to realize baseball might be the key to getting to know me. He tried, he really did. He took me to games and did his best to understand what was happening, but in the end it just wasn't for him. Neither was I. There was such a sweetness in his wanting to make it work badly enough to try to love what I loved alongside me, though. Mike, wherever you are, I will always respect you for that.

Eventually, I couldn't stand being separated from my home team, so I started to travel to see the Braves play in Denver and Phoenix. The Denver games I turned into a solo vacation, making new friends among my fellow fans in the hotel bar and chatting with the nicest usher ever about, of all things, the Chicago Cubs. The last year Chipper Jones played before his retirement I saw him play in Phoenix. The game capped off a weekend spent at the Pat Tillman memorial road race, again by myself, and again making new friends among fellow Braves fans at a bar. In a way it was lonely, but part of me relished the opportunity to get to the ballpark early for batting practice, study the program, and really focus on watching the game without any annoying distractions.

In August of 2012, on a random whim, I moved to San Diego. I had never even been there. Some strange voice just told me I needed to go. I was excited to be in a bigger city and, if not near my Braves, at least in a place with a major league park and the chance for my home team to come through and play at least once a year. I discovered once again that being a sports fan is a way to build a connection with people when you're new in town. One Saturday morning I walked into a bar to watch the Georgia Bulldogs play football with the alumni club and across the room, just grinning at me like a Cheshire cat, sat the man who would eventually become my husband.

As I got to know him, I realized that although we both happened to be in California, we had grown up in Georgia towns just a few miles apart and shared not only a love of Georgia football, but also a love of the Braves. When Shep and I first met, I was dating some other guy, and when that other guy

Baseball

stood me up for a date one night (Thanks, Kevin! No, really. I've been meaning to send a card), Shep took me to the batting cages to unleash all the angst. I got into the "fast" baseball cage and actually managed to make contact with a few pitches. That made me feel like a million bucks, but more importantly, it showed me that this guy understood the pathway to my soul.

By the time spring rolled around, we had realized we were meant to be together and we started taking advantage of the Padres season tickets I had ordered when I first moved to town. The first time we went to a game, he told me he liked to get to the stadium early to watch batting practice. My battered little heart grew about three sizes just hearing him say such a thing. Our home team came to town in May, and we got to see our favorite new player, Evan Gattis. We talked about our mutual childhood love of Dale Murphy and how no player had excited us the same way until Gattis came along. Gattis was old for a rookie. He had spent several years longer than most getting his life together, and his profile picture on Twitter was his employee badge from the janitorial company where he worked cleaning office buildings until he got his big break. We got close enough to the visitors' dugout before the game to toss Gattis some baseballs and our Braves hats, which he autographed. It was a real thrill to watch him play.

In 2013 we decided to move back to Georgia together. Seeing my family and old friends and having access to my favorite foods again were all positive things, but what I most looked forward to was getting to go to Braves games again. Walking back into Turner Field for the first time after all those years away was intensely joyful. The sights, sounds, and smells brought back all of my childhood memories, and getting to experience that with my soulmate was beyond description. All that time, as we grew up in separate towns, living separate lives, this Braves fandom was the thread that wove us together. We had both spent childhood summer nights falling asleep listening to the Braves on the radio. We had both recorded games from the radio on cassette tapes so we could listen to them to soothe us through the dark of winter. The Braves represented the best parts of our emotional bonds with our respective fathers.

To both of us, it was so much more than just a game. When people ask me why I own 500 different Braves jerseys, sweatshirts, hats, books, VHS tapes, bobble-head statues, ticket stubs, baseball cards, and little plastic helmets that used to be filled with stadium soft serve ice cream, well, it's because the Braves are part of the very fabric of who I am. They're my eternal connection to the people I love and to some of the ones I've lost along the way. They're my anchor to my hometown and my way of life. There are a lot of things in this world that keep us distant from one another, and I will never regret spending my time, money, and efforts on a beautiful pastime that binds us together.

MY LITTLE PONY: FRIENDSHIP IS MAGIC
"Things Everypony Wants to Know but Is Afraid to Ask"
by Melissa D. Aaron

As you've probably seen from other essays in this book, it's very common for fans of one thing to be involved in a few other fandoms. My own primary fandom is Harry Potter and many of my fellow Harry Potter fans are ardent Whovians, Sherlockians, or obsessed with Game of Thrones. Whenever someone asks what else I am into, I mention a few fandoms, and then I add, "...and of course, My Little Pony, Friendship is Magic. Cue the glazed-over eyes, the careful edge away.

It needn't be this way.

I'd like to start with a bit of what academics call "positionality," or, put more simply, where I come from into this fandom. In broad terms, most outsiders put adult pony fans in two separate categories. The first would be fans of the original toys and the show. Many of these are collectors; most of them are female. The second group consists of fans of the rebooted cartoon developed for television by Lauren Faust. This group—often called Bronies—is usually assumed to be almost entirely male. The assumption partly comes from media coverage: young men carrying around pink and rainbow pony plushies are violating a gender stereotype, and hence more interesting to write about. It also comes from the assumption that everyone on the internet is male. I have experienced extreme surprise when a fellow online MLP fan discovers that I'm a woman (quote: "you're a girl?!!!??") Yes, I'm a woman, and I watch a TV show with unicorns, rainbows, and tea parties. Who would have thought? Reading pony fan blogs, following artists, and scanning through pony fanfiction would reveal that there are many women in the Fandom.

I don't identify as a "Brony," mostly because I've never been a "bro" and don't intend to start now. I also didn't grow up with the cartoon or the pony toys because I'm too old. I was already headed for college when the first toys were hitting the market in the 1980s. These toys, strange as it may seem, were initially intended as a re-framing of girl's toys. Bonnie Zacherle, the original designer, based on her own childhood experiences, insisted that girls who couldn't have ponies of their own would love to have realistic colored ponies with brushable hair. These were not the miniaturized household implements little girls supposedly wanted. Zacherle was reluctantly convinced to allow the ponies to be made smaller and in pastel colors, because pink and purple focus-grouped well, and thus started the Great Pony Boom.

Some fans, regardless of gender, will insist that they like the show because it isn't "girly." This is a shame. It presumes that "girliness" is necessarily a bad thing. It was with some relief that I read Lauren Faust's foreword to The Elements of Harmony, in which she defends the supposed "frilly pink silliness" of little girls and their imaginations. The whole essay is worth a read, but here is a quote:

> Rainbows, unicorns, fairy tales, hearts, stars, cupcakes, and, of course, pretty pastel ponies. Many people look at these things and roll their eyes. They can't imagine there could be anything more to such things beyond what they appear to be. But not little girls. They know something that we do not...To a little girl...This. Stuff. Is. Serious. To her, magic is not frivolous and silly; it is huge, and it is glorious. It is real. In

My Little Pony

My Little Pony: Friendship is Magic, friendship is literally magic. It defeats evil by means of the Elements of Harmony: Laughter, Loyalty, Generosity, Kindness, Honesty, and Magic itself.

In the world of Harry Potter, the same kind of magic is referred to as Love: "the power that the Dark Lord knows not." See? It's deeper than you think.

From my own point of view, My Little Pony represents continuity, not rupture. I am a former little girl who still loves tea parties and big hats. I am the proud owner of at least one tiara, and I never gave up on girliness. Especially not the cupcakes. That said, I came to My Little Pony through a not-particularly-girly, cross-fandom source: an Avengers fanfic called, "I Used to Wonder What Friendship Could Be." All of the Avengers were secretly Bronies and dared not let any of the others know that they watched a little girl's cartoon: all of them except for Thor, who greets Loki with a hearty, "Brother! You have finally accepted my invitation to watch the brightly colored ponies with me!" How could I not follow up on this? I had been exposed to the Pony Virus, and was showing the first symptom: curiosity.

I watched a number of episodes, until I came to "Read It and Sleep." This episode contains a miniature Indiana Jones-like movie, complete with sepia color saturation and a John Williams-style score. The thought occurred to me: "This is really unnecessarily good." So many cartoons aimed exclusively at children really aren't very good: doubly so if the intended audience is female. This one, though, had an individual background score in every episode. It had pastiches of adventure film, film noir, and Sondheim musicals. And I quickly realized that it had the same essential message as Harry Potter, my primary fandom and true love.

I was hooked.

Melissa D. Aaron

My Little Pony intersects with a lot of different fandoms. Where there are no obvious intersections, such as Sondheim musicals or *Star Trek* references, the fandom creates them. One of the most popular crossover characters began as a simple brown background pony with a spiky brown mane and an hourglass cutie mark on his flank. He was quickly dubbed Doctor Whooves, and became the star of many fanworks. Hasbro and the creators at the studio, DHX, have become aware of the passions of the adult fandom, and is willing to indulge them, within reason. Licensed T shirts of the Doctor began to appear, then Funko Pops, until finally the Doctor himself made an appearance in Episode 100, a splashy bit of crossover fanservice called "Slice of Life," in which the dreams of many, many Bronies came true.

A few other crossover elements include Twilight Sparkle wearing a number "42" in a race and saying ominously, "winter is coming." The ambiguously villainous chaos monster Discord closely resembles Q from *Star Trek: The Next Generation*, and is voiced by Q's actor, John de Lancie. The first two seasons draw heavily on Harry Potter. I have sometimes described the show as "Harry Potter, if there was no Harry, and Hermione was a purple unicorn." Both include a mentor who leaves his or her student to deal with existential threats, and then comes back, explains everything, and twinkles. Princess Celestia even has a phoenix for a pet. Essentially, she is Dumbledore, only with pastel rainbow hair, and a lot more fabulous. Her younger sister, Luna, who rules the night as Celestia rules the day, has a chariot, drawn, apparently, by Thestrals. The attempted Lord of the Rings crossover didn't work quite as well. Even with ponies miserably chained together like the slaves of Barad-Dur, it's hard to create the pony version of Sauron. In general, there's lots of pop cultural references to draw in fans from other fandoms.

My Little Pony

One attraction for me was that the show passes the Bechdel test in every episode. The main characters are all female, and they are all very different, from the athletic braggart Rainbow Dash to the tremulous animal-lover Fluttershy. Faust said that she intentionally created a show that would demonstrate that there were many different ways of being a girl. Romantic relationships are downplayed or non-existent. This is what I had to do to find a show with a large female cast that was not focused on sex or romance: I had to find it in a cartoon for little girls. That's how hard it was. Fortunately, it still hasn't been cancelled for being "too female." In the earlier seasons, there were almost no important male characters. Different fans interpreted this in different ways, and some complained about it, but I simply assumed that Equestria was something like Wonder Woman's Themiscyra, and I liked it.

Harry Potter has often been accused, wrongly, of teaching witchcraft, but I've been surprised that My Little Pony, with its princesses responsible for raising the sun and the moon by magic, and who have been ruling for well over a thousand years, hasn't been accused of goddess-centered Paganism. Like Wonder Woman, problems with other sapient beings are usually worked out with friendship or peace as a first attempt, with toned-down cartoon violence only used as a last resort.

Hugs and cupcakes are the essence of the show, and I don't think that's a bad thing.

Stereotypically "girly" characters and plots have been re-worked. Rarity, the pony who is fascinated by fashion, is not a shopper, but a designer who works at making her visions reality, obsessed with perfection. The shy little animal-lover pegasus Fluttershy has the Doolittle-ish ability to speak with animals and tells off dragons when she has to. And one of the oldest, most hackneyed plots of little girl cartoons, the "why aren't my friends coming to my party?" plot, has been rewritten so that its cute little pink pony main character, Pinkie Pie, has a total psychotic meltdown when her friends don't show. So closely identified with parties and making other ponies happy is she that she cannot face the situation, and instead throws a party for a bag of flour, a pile of rocks, and a bucket of turnips. She is a terror to behold. It's quite subversive. This episode, "Party of One," almost requires the analytical experience of little girls to decode. The emotional response to being rejected by friends is not gentle weeping into a party napkin. It is rage. And it's important to control that rage and give your friends a chance to explain themselves (and, in this case, to throw you a surprise party). Despite this alarming episode, Pinkie Pie is, as pony fans say, Best Pony.

MLP also has a number of spinoffs, most notably the comic books published by IDW. This has become the source of many "is it or isn't it canon" arguments. Personally, I wouldn't want to miss them, as they add all kinds of things not covered in the show, such as the secretly tragic love life of Princess Celestia. At least, unlike Dumbledore, she had one, right?

So how do I personally geek out? Naturally, as a fanfic writer, I gravitated toward fanfiction. There are two major online venues for MLP fanfic. One is Equestria Daily, the primary source of MLP news, gossip, analysis, and heavily curated art in multiple forms. The other is a site dedicated exclusively to MLP fanfiction, FiMFiction. There are many writers' groups, groups specializing in certain characters or ships, and review groups that review select relatively little known fanworks. I initially intended to write a few amusing little fanfics. Almost 200,000 words later...

My Little Pony

There are other fanworks I don't produce, but simply consume and enjoy. The MLP fandom has many talented artists and musicians. I have a workout playlist with a high intensity segment: the songs "Simply Dashing," by M. Pallante, inspired by Rainbow Dash, and "Never Back Down," by the Aviators, similarly inspired by Dash's favorite fictional character, Daring Do. I'm not much of an athlete, but I don't like letting Dashie down, and I find that I push myself just a bit harder. It's easy to get lost in MLP-inspired artwork, although it's wise to enable Safe Search on the browser, just in case.

I suspect most fans create artificial lines in the sand, past which they tell themselves they will not go. "I will not go to a midnight showing. I will not attend a convention. I will not cosplay. I will not cosplay anything I have to make myself while wearing a respirator. I will neither draw fanart nor write fanfiction, and if I do, I will not put it online," etc. I have blown past nearly all of these, but I can come up with some very good excuses.

Attending MLP conventions didn't seem to be that big of a deal. I live in the Greater Los Angeles area, where there are many fan conventions within an easy drive. It only made sense to go to EQLA, and it was well worth it to go to panels with the show's musicians and browse the vendor's room. After all, I wasn't wearing ears or wings or anything. Since I'd gone once, I might as well go again, right? Several years later, EQLA brought Zacherle and Faust together, where they met onstage and in real life for the first time. It was a great generational moment.

I'm glad I was there.

BabsCon, in the Bay Area, wasn't all that far away, comparatively speaking, and there were things I wanted to do there. Also, I had created a really good Cherry Jubilee cosplay by then, and I wanted to be seen. I suppose it was only a matter of time before I wound up on a fanfiction panel at BronyCon, at which male writers outnumbered female writers four to two: a panel discussing something I definitely had said I wouldn't do.

I began with the firm conviction that I would not ship ponies. After all, one of the pleasures of MLP is that it has very few canon ships. It doesn't have romance. It doesn't need it. It's extremely rare to find a show that has a large female cast which is plot focused and not derailed by love interests. It was a refuge, so I was adamantly on the side of not shipping ponies. Then the episode "Pinkie Pride" aired, and I did a complete 180. To my embarrassment, I began shipping Pinkie and Cheese Sandwich—a character voiced by Weird Al Yankovic—like crazy. They obviously belonged together. This is how I wrote those 200,000 words and wound up on that BronyCon panel: a panel about shipping and writing romance fiction for ponies. I was now Horse Famous, as the Brony term goes, for writing shipfics. Oh, the shame.

Pony cosplay, and I have no shame about this, is tricky. The characters are ponies and not human, at least until recently, and this required either investing a fur suit, a length to which most fans won't go, or creating some sort of human approximation of that pony for cosplay purposes. The results can be extremely imaginative, especially since the characters themselves sometimes cross over into other franchises. How, for example, does one cosplay as Radiance, who is Rarity as a superhero? How does one dress as a humanized version of a unicorn reminiscent of Star Sapphire?

I chose Cherry Jubilee, a very minor one shot character, for two reasons: there weren't that many people who did a Cherry Jubilee cosplay, and she was the only female character of a certain age who wasn't somebody's mom.

My Little Pony

Cherry Jubilee's design is clearly modeled after Miss Kitty from Gunsmoke, so I created a saloon girl dress. It was the most complicated cosplay I have ever created, made of yards and yards of red and white silk taffeta. I am not kidding when I say that you could get married in that dress. This should have been a clue that I was getting a bit involved.

Pony customization is amazing to watch. The first custom pony I ever bought was a crossover Remus Lupin pony I acquired at a Harry Potter convention and promptly christened My Little Remus. I have nothing but admiration for those who painstakingly soak, dye, paint, and rehair ponies. It's something I personally wouldn't try, because you have to pop off their tiny heads, and I don't have the fortitude for this. Styling their hair, on the other hand, is addictive. Plastic ponies out of the pack don't match their show counterparts, and it's curiously absorbing to put their nylon hair in tiny perm rods, especially very late at night. Mine are also now signed by the voice artists.

For me, the final line in the sand was, "I will not commission a custom plushie." My Little Pony custom plushies can be incredibly expensive. Possibly the most expensive was a large Rainbow Dash; the final bid was close to 2,500. My BPFF (Best Pony Friend Forever), Elric of Melnipony, has suggested sardonically that they must be stuffed with gold dust and cocaine. In fairness to the plushie makers, the materials, especially the minky fabric, are not cheap. The patterns are frequently original, as are special techniques for decoration and hair, and they take many hours to make. A good pony plushie is a work of art. Still, they're awfully expensive, so I would never, ever...

...The two I have now are very nice plushies! They're a matched set! How many Rainbow Power Pinkie Pie plushies do you see, let alone a Cheese Sandwich complete with serape, hat, and rubber chicken! They are very beautiful, and I enjoyed the brainstorming with the plushie artist, who uses mohair for more life-like hair, rather than big pieces of fabric cut into show accurate shapes. The Rainbow Power Pinkie might be unique, and I don't care if I'm the only person who liked the design in the first place. They occupy their own glass-fronted cabinet, along with the autographed ponies, and I'm very proud of them.

I've been through most of the great fandom dramas that television fandoms seem to attract. I started watching the show after the infamy that was Derpygate, but I watched as the fandom melted down over the introduction of an unsuspected brother of Twilight Sparkle and a third alicorn (unicorns with wings: princesses by definition in Equestria). 2013 was a particularly rough year, as it included the introduction of humanized, high school versions of the ponies ("Equestria Girls,") and also the ascension of Twilight Sparkle to Princesshood, accompanied by the sudden growth of wings. Curiously, the scene in which this happens is strongly reminiscent of the King's Cross chapter of Harry Potter and the Deathly Hallows, in which the main character's mentor reviews the life and the choices of the protagonist and asserts his or her pride in the younger character. Harry doesn't grow wings or become a princess, but even so, the parallels are remarkable.

Eventually, the fandom absorbed these changes, as fandoms tend to do, but emotions run high. Frequently, the bursts of unhappiness over more princesses, Breezies, human high school ponies, and—soon—sea ponies,

My Little Pony

seem based in the complaint that the show is too "toyetic," that, in fact, it has its roots in a cartoon for little girls and the imaginative stories they make up with their toy ponies. I believe that this is where we came in.

So, really, that's why I geek out over My Little Pony. It lets me access that little girl again: a clever, imaginative, emotionally rich little girl, who still loves unicorns, rainbows, and cupcakes, especially the cupcakes.

And girly is ok.

Girly is good.

THE WEST WING, BREAKING BAD, & TWIN PEAKS
"Not a Nerdtypical Response"
by Cat Smith

I was at a nerd function recently, chatting with a friend of mine about some of the things we consider iconic in current Nerd World. We talked about *Doctor Who*, and *Game of Thrones*, and *Wonder Woman*. And then I mentioned *Breaking Bad* – and she said something like, "but that doesn't really count".

And I wondered why. Why does something like *Breaking Bad* not get to exist as easily in a conversation about "nerd loves" as something like *Star Wars*? It can't be because it's popular – *Star Wars* is more popular than ever nowadays. It can't be because it takes place in the real world – the world of Walter White isn't any more "real" than the world of Diana Prince. It isn't because non-nerds also love it – *Game of Thrones* is a huge crossover hit, beloved by nerds and mainstream fans alike. And *Game of Thrones* gets its share of Emmys, so it can't be critical acclaim. I was baffled. I still am.

I love my nerd family. I truly do. Nerd World will love you when no one else does. That said, I'm still a bit of an outsider – a weirdo among weirdos. Full disclosure – I'm not huge with the sci-fi/fantasy. I didn't get on the *Doctor Who* bandwagon until 2011. I don't care about superheroes, and I'm kind of over most Disney. I go to New York Comic Con with my badge hanging off my *Newsroom* lanyard, and I'm pretty sure that is the only piece of *Newsroom* merch in the joint. Nerds are my people... but even more my people are the subset of nerds who exist within Nerd World but are not "nerdtypical". (Is nerdtypical a word? It is now.) I love my nerdtypical stuff, and my cosplay, and my Funko Pops, but let me talk to you for a minute about the things I love more.

The West Wing

First of all, you have to know – I am not politically minded and never have been. Every election cycle I have to do a crash course in candidates so that I can be vaguely informed when I show up to vote (hey, I said I wasn't political. I never said I was irresponsible.) I never, not in a million years, would have thought I would give a crap about the inner workings of any White House, real or fictional. I would absolutely never have thought I would enjoy watching a television show about said workings. "Not my genre," I said, and I said it to many – friends, relatives, maybe even strangers. Anyone who tried to tell me, "no seriously – you should try this, you will like it, honest."

I was diagnosed with Multiple Sclerosis (MS) in 2003. We found it early and I'm fine, thanks, but suddenly, those well-intentioned masses started in with their recommendations again, now with a spoiler as well – now I REALLY needed to watch *The West Wing*, because "their President has MS and it's really interesting and I should watch it." I said, "Are you all crazy? Having told me this, I should absolutely NOT watch this show, for the same reasons hypochondriacs shouldn't watch *House*." The last thing I needed to see was some fictional person exhibiting symptoms that I may or may not have, because both my brain and body hate me (and I promise you I will start exhibiting those symptoms once I know they are a possibility). The resistance continued – though I had to admit, the thought of someone with the same condition as me, running the country (presumably with way more stress), was comforting. I didn't want to watch the show, but I thought Aaron Sorkin had done a cool thing in writing it, and I mentioned around that it would be cool to say thank you to him.

Cut to about 5 years later. Aaron Sorkin has been commissioned to write a screenplay about Facebook. Figuring that he ought to actually know something about Facebook, he gets a public page, and for a long time, he is a terribly good sport about questions and discussions. An old friend let me know about the existence of this page and I jumped – "Dear Mister Sorkin, I don't watch your show and I don't ever plan to, because hypochondriacs and *House*, but the thought of this does my heart good, and probably other MS-havers as well, so thanks." He wrote back right away, and told me I knocked his socks off.

Well, that's enough to warm anyone up to something, don't you think? My summer job takes me to a camp in the Catskills where I don't get TV service, so my clever brother (who was a big fan already) simply handed me the DVDs, knowing I would get bored in the evenings and succumb. By the way, to round out the Aaron story, I went back to the Facebook page to tell him I had changed my mind and was watching the show. It was ten months later and he remembered who I was, greeted me like an old friend, and even gave me a heads up on two of the more MS-heavy episodes that might upset me ("He Shall, From Time To Time…" and "17 People"— he wasn't wrong). He was also impressed that I spotted one of what he considered one of his more obscure Gilbert and Sullivan references – it is wonderful to watch television that is written by people who are musical theatre nerds… at least, for me it is. I didn't think the reference was that obscure.

The show is really about smart people. Smart people saying smart things and saying those things really, really fast. Smart people being super capable and professional at their jobs, and yet ridiculously human, and often quite awkward. I'm not so much into comedies, where the whole point of the show is to make you laugh, and that's what they are working for – I like wit, and real plots, involving people who happen to have senses of humour. I relate to that. This show was built on that. Most importantly, I LIKED these people. Every single one of them. This was a group of well-intentioned, hardworking people trying to make the world a better place, and I admired them for it. I don't think there was a single member of that White House staff that I didn't want to hug at some point. As Sam Seaborn, Rob Lowe is his ridiculously pretty self, only it doesn't matter because he doesn't "know how to girl" at all and he is so brilliant that his being pretty becomes the least of what he is. As Leo McGarry, John Spencer is crusty and unflappable, a man who still wrestles his demons every day, respects the hell out of them, but has made them his bitch. And as Jed Bartlet, Martin Sheen is the President that every well-read, loquacious, nerd dreams of having in the White House. I could go on and on.

I have to give CJ Cregg her own paragraph here. Allison Janney being a brilliant actress aside (yes, continue to shower this woman with Emmys, please), I think CJ is one of the greatest female characters ever written. I've got a small handful of friends who refer to me as the CJ in their lives, and to me, that's some of the highest possible praise, of which I am hardly worthy. CJ is a woman in a man's job, in one of the ultimate boys' clubs (Washington is becoming more integrated all the time, but it is a slow road), and she is tough and smart and sassy and holds her own with the boys, while all the while looking smashing in her Vera Wang, working through her (extremely funny) root canal, or having to endure the First Lady trying to set her up with cardiologists. Even Janney talks unendingly about what a role model CJ is for herself – though, Sorkin credits Janney for most of the character, so you have to wonder which of them is being more falsely modest. It has always frustrated me when Aaron Sorkin gets criticized for his so-called sexism – I think CJ (and Abbey Bartlet, and Ainsley Hayes, and Dolores Landingham, and half the women he's written) are proof that he is an absolute feminist ally. Maybe he is a little blinded by his own gender perspective, but he is definitely one of the good guys.

Sure, *The West Wing* is an idealized view of the political situation, and I would guess that real politics is probably closer to the *House of Cards* side of the equation (*shudder*). But you know what? Apart from being clever, and witty, and charming, and engaging, and entertaining, the show is also comforting. It gives me hope that if one man could imagine a vision like this, maybe others could too, and maybe some of those people could work toward making the world better in real life. Nowadays, I know I am, and many others are, rewatching the show as a refuge from the disturbing real life political climate. And I'll tell you something – the world would definitely be a better place if all Republicans were Sorkin Republicans. Even though the Bartlet White House is a Democratic White House, rarely are Republicans simply THE BAD GUYS – they have a different view, and most of them are willing to talk rationally. Arnie Vinick? Please. Could real life have its own Arnie Vinick? Or Ainsley Hayes? For all the jokes that she is "slightly to the right of the Kaiser", I find myself quoting her in countless discussions regarding not only politics, but feminism.

I like to learn things, even if it's by accident. It's no wonder to me that teenagers tell me that *The West Wing* is shown to them in school by their government or social studies teachers. If *West Wing* had existed when I was in school, my grades would have been a lot better. And *West Wing* quotes provide me with ammunition for half the debates I get into, about anything. To say nothing of the many ways quotes from this show have casually worked their way into my everyday vocabulary (probably making me seem smarter and wittier than I am), or how the word "okay" can, in the right hands, hide a paragraph's worth of meaning behind two syllables.

The West Wing taught me this very important lesson – if the writing is THAT good, then genre doesn't matter. And the writing is THAT good. When I poked my head out of mainstream nerd world, and looked beyond the Buffy and Star Wars fans that made up most of my friend base, lo and behold, it turned out that some of the people I got along with best happened to be fans of *The West Wing* too – but this fandom kind of got overshadowed by the more nerdtypical, colourful shows. After all, there aren't all that many cosplay possibilities in The West Wing unless you are lucky enough to look like one of the actors, and when something is as much of a mainstream success as this was, winning Emmy after Emmy, it is easy to disassociate it from the shows that are normally discussed on con panels. I happened to have enough street cred with the showrunners of New York based con LI Geek that I was able to host two successful panels about the Sorkin television shows – but such a thing is largely unheard of. Sure, we have our own hand signal, but in my circles we Sorkinites are the weirdos in a superhero-loving world. And truly, I've never met anyone who, having watched the show (and I mean properly watched it, not just caught an episode here or there) thinks it is anything short of wonderful.

Cat Smith

A thousand blessings on Lin-Manuel Miranda, my favourite fanboy, and how his unashamed groupie-ness of *The West Wing* was hugely inspirational in his writing of *Hamilton: An American Musical*, which has its own enormous following and has won pretty much every award on the planet (at his last performance in the title role, his final curtain call was televised, and the orchestra surprised him by playing the *West Wing* theme). *Doctor Who's* Tenth Doctor, David Tennant, my second favourite fanboy, is also a great big *West Wing* nerd. To the extent of appearing in a British quiz show that was produced when the series ended – it's called "The Ultimate West Wing Challenge", and you can find it on YouTube, and see Tennant and the other contestants spewing out trivia that even I think is obscure. And for round two, in the spirit of the famous Aaron Sorkin/Tommy Schlamme "walk-and-talk", they put the contestants on treadmills which gradually speed up as the trivia questions get harder.

I've seen convention photos that *Doctor Who* fans have paid large amounts of money for, and there's David Tennant, photobombing the *Doctor Who* experience with his *West Wing* tee shirt (I love him more for this). There is also a whole book that was compiled by Claire Handscombe, *Walk With Us: How "The West Wing" Changed Our Lives,* it is people telling their stories about how this show changed their lives, woke them up, inspired them to change themselves, and change the world. (I'm in it.) People have even gone into politics because of this show. A community of people dedicated to changing the world... if that doesn't count as fandom, I don't know what does.

The West Wing, Breaking Bad, & Twin Peaks

Breaking Bad

Let me tell you something, there are worse reasons to watch a show than parental bonding. As with *The West Wing*, I shied away from *Breaking Bad* because I had no interest in the premise, but it was a favourite of my dad's, and he kept nudging me. I don't know about you, but something else you can have conversations with your father about is only ever a good thing. Besides, we both loved *The Newsroom* and *Game of Thrones*, so it's not like our tastes were alien to each other. And I knew *Breaking Bad* was laden with Emmys, and lots of people were crazy for it, so I finally said what the hell and started watching.

I'm not going to lie, I wasn't grabbed right away. I wasn't sure I could like Walter White, and it took me a little while to realise that I didn't really need to do so. The idea of a villain protagonist in television isn't something I was used to – and with Walt, he's that frog in the boiling water whose evil sneaks up on you before you know what's going on. It's the main thing I love about the characters on this show – everybody's complicated. I may not agree with every choice that Skyler White makes, but I understand them. It took me two rewatches to appreciate the complex mastery that is Hank Schrader, but now I love him to the moon and back. And you want to talk smart, and well-crafted, and gorgeous cinematography – well, pretty soon the show made me its bitch, and I could see what everyone else had been raving about. Just like with *The West Wing*, the writing was THAT good, so I didn't care anymore about the premise. I also find that *Breaking Bad* has affected my casual speech a great deal, similar to *The West Wing* – though in this case, it presents itself in excessive uses of the words "yo" and "bitch".

So, I can't really claim this show has been good for my vocabulary the way Sorkin has, but there it is.

The *Breaking Bad* fan experience is a strange one for me, and not just because it is outside the zone of the nerdtypical. I mean, unlike *The West Wing*, you could go to Comicon and buy as much merch as you please. You might even come across a Walter White cosplayer or two (I had great success when my boyfriend and I mashed up a *Breaking Bad/Doctor Who* team cosplay – "Breaking Bad Wolf". (I figure, Rose and Metacrisis Ten had to earn a living in the parallel dimension, right? So maybe the TARDIS cooks really good meth. But I digress). But all of this is outside the zone. You won't find a cosplay group, and if there's a discussion panel, odds are good that I'm the one running it.

Being a female *Breaking Bad* fan is sometimes problematic. I can't tell you how many times I have suggested the show to female friends when they request suggestions of what to watch next and have gotten told "yeah, but that's a BOY show". They're not entirely wrong. The only female cosplayers you see are usually sexy femme!Walt and Jesse, and I've seen girls dressed as bags of blue meth. Once, online, I saw a girl dressed as Lydia, and I want to meet and hug this girl. I cosplay Skyler, and dammit, I am going to get underwater photos one of these days – but right there is why female fandom of this show is sometimes hard, and why I felt the need to cosplay Skyler in her pool outfit.

Breaking Bad is centered on such a male power fantasy, and if you are a fan of that fantasy (which the lion's share of the fandom is), Skyler is the main obstacle to that fantasy. It is ridiculous how much hate for not only the character but also the actress is all over the internet (come on, people, learn to separate an actor from their JOB, okay?), and it makes me angry and sad. I hate to say it about a show I love, because it certainly isn't the show's fault, but I have found there is a river of misogyny that runs through the fandom. I am absolutely not saying that every Breaking Bad fan I meet is a sexist pig, but there is a lot of it out there (some of it accidental, some not), and Skyler bears the brunt of it. I'm not here to debate that, but I will just say that if I didn't love Skyler anyway, I would support the crap out of her on principle. I'm a contrary cuss in my fandoms (and in life, really) – I have a tendency to back the underdog. I've even seen female fans bashing her, which baffles me. I think the support of Skyler White (or at least, the defense of her) is kind of crucial in nerd fandom, where strong women who don't wield swords, stakes, or chakrams are woefully underrepresented.

To dismiss Skyler as a bitch (or Hank as a loud, obnoxious guy – which he is, no question, but he is so much more than that) is to turn your back on a huge part of what makes *Breaking Bad* so incredible. It is absolutely valid to like a show simply because it is shiny and pretty and exciting, and *Breaking Bad* is certainly that. But if you want to fully appreciate its genius, and why (like *The West Wing*) it got Emmy after Emmy thrown at it, you have to look beneath the surface – even if you are content with just the surface. That's what I like in my television, though I know it's not a common attitude. And that point brings me to –

Twin Peaks

I'm *Twin Peaks* OG – I was 18 or so when it aired, and I was one of those people who huddled round their televisions on Thursday nights, barely breathing until the commercials. And obsessing the way we had to in the primordial soup of the pre-internet world – in person, or over the phone, to (*gasp!*) one person at a time. That summer when we were waiting to find out if Agent Cooper had been wearing a bulletproof vest or not was the longest three months of my young life. We had fanzines instead of chat rooms. We had weekly parties for the new episodes, complete with coffee, donuts, and pie.

As of this writing, it is 2017, and we are about a third of the way into *Twin Peaks: The Return*, courtesy of Showtime. When it was first announced on Twitter two years ago, the explosion shook the internet. All of a sudden, this weird, quirky show that I had rewatched yearly ever since the first VHS tapes became available was hugely popular again, and to a whole new generation of fans. People who weren't even alive when the show first aired were running to Netflix to binge-watch it, creating Facebook discussion groups, and buying plaid skirts so they can cosplay Audrey Horne.

On the one hand, that's fantastic. It's great fun to re-live this show that I have loved for years through fresh eyes, and I'm glad that it is part of the national consciousness again. On the other hand, I can't help feeling a little possessive about it – kid, some of us have been waiting for this LONGER THAN YOU HAVE BEEN ALIVE *shakes fist at swinging traffic light – err... cloud*. We didn't have Netflix! We didn't have the INTERNET, for god's sake! You don't know how important this really is! I was watching the premiere with some friends, all of whom were a lot younger than me and when one of them got choked up over the appearance of the Log Lady, I got irrationally angry. I kept it to myself, of course, but in my head I was going "you've seen every episode exactly ONCE! Two measly years ago! You haven't earned those tears!"

The West Wing, Breaking Bad, & Twin Peaks

Which, of course, is a dumb way to feel, which is why I didn't say anything – there's enough of that attitude going around in the *Doctor Who* community, and it's dumb there too. There's no wrong way to be a fan (unless your fan-ness is to the detriment of others, in which case you are actual fandom trash – don't get me started on that expression, here's hoping it dies out by the time this is published). Who really cares if you are late to the party – it's great that you finally made it! But honestly (and I'm not proud of this), it gave me an irrational sympathy for the people who complain about cultural appropriation. *Twin Peaks*, in all its weird and wacky glory, has been my culture, and you are appropriating it!

Let me reiterate – those feelings are dumb and irrational, and I'm truly happy that *The Return* exists, and is bringing more people into the Lynch fold. It seems to be doing well, though there is always that breed of *Twin Peaks* fan who didn't like *Fire – Walk With Me* (FWWM) because it was such a departure from the series, and since *The Return* is on cable and doesn't have to cater to Standards and Practices, the tone of it is a lot closer to *FWWM* than it is to the network series. I myself love *FWWM* even though it's different. I mean, the very first image that you see after the opening credits is a television being smashed. If that isn't a clear message of "this ain't yo mama's *Twin Peaks*", I don't know what is. I get that we all wanted to know what happened after the series ended on such a cliffhanger. I wanted to know what happened too.

FWWM didn't answer any of those questions – it was a prequel, and we knew what was going to happen. People complained, especially if they hadn't read Laura's diary (which, if you ask me, should have been handed out as homework before you were even allowed to buy your ticket to the film). It's always interesting to see how audiences evolve, and what different things become important over the years. A friend of mine recently saw *FWWM* for the first time, and she remarked that she doesn't understand the haters of Laura's story – that if a lifetime of sexual abuse is not more important to you than the owls not being what they seem, your priorities are seriously out of whack. And she was right, of course – but that's not something we noticed at the time. At least I didn't – but I loved the film right at the off.

As stated, I've watched the original series at least every couple of years since it aired. It's this many years later, and I'm still noticing new things (all those *Glass Menagerie* references? Did you catch those?). People are going to be talking about *The Return* 25 years from now. I haven't been (yet), but there is a yearly *Twin Peaks* Fest that takes place in the town where they shot the exteriors – it's a proper con, with guests, cosplay, panels, and everything – and I bet you ticket sales are going to skyrocket. *Twin Peaks* has always kind of been its own weird subset of fandom – it's not a total mainstream crossover like *Breaking Bad*, nor is it among the nerdtypical. Twin Peaks paved the way for things like *Lost* and *Mad Men*, and now I have to wonder if those shows (that were huge mainstream hits) helped pave the way for *The Return* to be able to happen. It's a beautiful example of media integration – the blurred lines between the nerdypical and the mainstream successes. And that is kind of the point I was originally trying to make – that nothing "doesn't really count". If lots of people love it, it's a fandom, for better or for worse.

AGENT CARTER
"I Know My Value"
by Scarlett Jaye

"I know my value."

I begin every day now with that thought in my mind and that quote on my lips; my mornings begin with me declaring "I know my value" as surely as every faerie tale begins with "Once upon a time".

Once upon a time, there was a little girl who, try as she might, could not relate to the other little girls. While they played princesses, she played knights of the roundtable; while they played supermodel, she played superhero; while they went to school dances, she went to the comic book store.

Predictably, that little girl was me, and should I ever find a DeLorean or a TARDIS or a path across the Bifrost, I would go back to that little girl, sitting alone on a swing in the park, kneel in front of her, and tell her, "It will all be all right. The things that make you different today will find you friends in the future; there will be laughter and adventure; there will be celebrations of heroes." And when she would ask me, "Who are you?" I would reply, "Why, I'm you; you will see."

I distinctly remember one day when I wore my school shoes and stockings out to play after school and the other children mocked me. In a completely misguided attempt to comfort me, a playmate began giving me "advice" as to how to "fit in", and then said the worst, most condescending thing I could imagine: "I used to be just like you."

Scarlett Jaye

I believe that was the first time it had occurred to me that someone thought being *me* was *bad*. I had never thought of such a possibility before, and I didn't like it. I can remember other instances— my entire gym class teasing me about the brand new sneakers my father had bought for me for my first year of high school (someone even signed my yearbook four years later mocking them); a girl magnanimously offering to flat iron my hair on a freshman year trip because my hair was frizzy and wavy— more indicators that being *me* was something that needed *changing*.

Nowadays, I stride out of my apartment dressed in 1940s-style dresses, blouses, skirts and shoes. I love a good hat. I have been lucky enough to learn how to do a 1940s pin curl set from trained hair and wig stylists and for the first time I am embracing my curly brown hair and feeling glamorous. People stop me on the streets of New York to tell me how much they like my dresses. I had a girl ask for my photo because she was doing a research paper on vintage dressing in modern New York and she exclaimed, "You're exactly what my paper is about!" I have had tourists on Broadway ask me if I was in "the show" (*War Paint* was playing and I couldn't ask for a better compliment). I felt happy tears springing to my eyes just recently because a friend told me, "I just realized who it is you look like – Rita Hayworth."

I couldn't imagine a more flattering person to be compared to than Miss Hayworth. And this is all because Peggy Carter showed me there's more than one way to dress – that I didn't have to take the advice of that long-ago playmate who was just trying to convince me to look like everyone else. That I could be pretty *my* way, the way *I* wanted to be.

What a thrill to be stopped on the street and complimented. What magic to be told I look like an old Hollywood pin-up. Especially for a girl like me – who had let the rejections from boys and the teasing from peers chip away at my self-esteem to the point where I was running nine miles a day and eating nothing but wedges of cheese to stay slim, to be liked, to be wanted. Unfortunately, that destructive behavior was rewarded with attention – from women who wanted to be me, and men who wanted to be with me. But I was still that scared little girl.

I got married mostly out of fear; fear of being alone, fear that no one else would want me, and fear that the first man who asked for my hand would be the best I could ever do. It was not a good marriage, and I was unhappy, but too scared and embarrassed to admit I might have made a mistake, that I might have let my fear drive me into something that wasn't right for me.

I still didn't know my value.

In the summer of 2015, my life as I knew it was completely destroyed. I moved from New York, my home, and left a job I loved dearly to live with my then-husband in his hometown some states over. Two weeks later, my deeply troubled then-husband had a very public nervous breakdown, threatened suicide, was arrested, and sent to the hospital. Upon his release, he left me and began divorce proceedings. Many mutual friends who didn't know the whole story (I refused and still refuse to disclose the worst parts; it was no one's business but mine and it would have felt like fighting dirty or trading on it to get sympathy) pitied my ex and showered him with attention while I, the woman who he had claimed he wanted to spend his life with, and who had spent years in the company of those friends, spent the rest of the year feeling like a calendar page that had been ripped off and thrown away.

Of course I was heartbroken. All in the span of a month, I lost my home, my job, my social circle, the man I had thought was my "Right Partner", and the life and future I had been so sure of. I lost my apartment lease and had to move in with my parents in a remote, isolated town far away from everyone and everything I cared about. I was extremely depressed, lonely, and confused, and I had lost all sense of self-worth. I questioned every decision I had ever made – I questioned my value, my beauty, my strength, my ability to love and to be loved. I thought that I would die there. Sometimes, on the worst days, I even wished I would.

Along with feeling abandoned and humiliated, my heart broken and my self-esteem crushed to powder, I had almost no social life. I had few phone calls or letters and even fewer visitors, so I watched a lot of movies and read a lot of comics to pass the time while saving up money to move back to Brooklyn, which will always be home to me. And it was there that I found Peggy Carter, first in the reels of *Captain America: The First Avenger* and then on television in *Agent Carter.* In those moments I was reminded I was not alone in how I felt. That maybe, just maybe, there was more out there for me.

Now, my ex-husband is no Steve Rogers. Not even close. In the end he was not heroic, or loving, or even kind. But Peggy has experienced loss and has experienced not just having to start all over again, but having to do it in a place where people who know a bit of her past give her wary looks. ("She wouldn't trade a red white and blue shield for a metal crutch.") Or they expect her to simply straighten up and act like it didn't happen. ("You used to be fun, Carter.") Or, they treat her like a spare part, someone to be disrespected and dismissed. ("Carter – man the phones.")

Agent Carter

I saw a lot of myself in that first season of her show – of trying to simply soldier on and let things go, the best you can, with seemingly constant opposition. I watched her do all that and be her own hero, and when she told Jarvis "I know my value," I am not ashamed to say I got a little teary-eyed.

Cosplay had been a huge part of my life as well as a huge part of my relationship with my ex-husband, and I had been hesitant to even put on my old costumes, unsure I could handle the memories. But thanks to Peggy, I sallied forth again, and my first cosplay after the divorce was Agent Carter, in her military uniform, just as she appeared in her first scene in *Captain America: The First Avenger*. It was not a particularly stellar costume, and I've made many improvements on it since then, along with amassing quite a few different costumes and looks for Peggy, but it was that critical first step that made me brave enough to put myself back out in that arena. Dressing up as Peggy that first time made me feel pretty and strong again – valuable – in the wake of that series of events after which I believed I could never feel that way again.

There is a wonderful scene in the first season of *Agent Carter* in which Peggy sits down to her first dinner at the boarding-house with her friend Angie. She meets the other residents, a group of women who immediately welcome Peggy into their circle, telling her how to sneak things past the house mother and smuggle food to squirrel away. One girl proudly shows off her new jumper in which her mother has knitted a "special chicken pocket". Peggy, who is initially hesitant to warm up to the women due to the dangerous nature of her work, cannot help but smile.

I've sat around similar tables, with my "agents"— a group of women I've met through cosplay, through fandom, through Peggy; women who have wonderful stories of their own to tell and things to teach. I've learned about sewing, about fashion, about hair styling, and these women share their knowledge with the best intentions and hearts of gold. There is an entire community of women who cosplay Peggy Carter out there, and I am proud to be a part of that community and call each and every one of them friends. I have made several incredibly strong friendships through the mutual admiration and respect for Peggy and what she teaches us, and I speak to these wonderful women and men every day; I can't imagine my life without them. A huge part of *Agent Carter* is the theme of women supporting and respecting each other--even the adversarial relationships between Dottie Underwood and Madame Masque and Peggy are built on respect, and I feel that respect every time I reach my arms out to accept a hug from the friends I've made through cosplay and fandom. I feel it every time they dry my tears or tell me they love me or push me to do my best. They make me feel every day that being *me* is not bad, that it is wonderful and special and *necessary* to be me, to be the best version of myself possible.

Peggy Carter has experienced loss. She has experienced hardship, and betrayal, and dismissal, and everyone throwing roadblocks in her way. She never gives up, even when it must feel like she's lost everything, even when it seems like every hand is turned against her.

There was one truly bleak night, out there in the middle of nowhere, in which I thought of drawing a bath, setting my hair, and simply ending it all. But I distinctly remember, alone in the house with only the cat for company, hearing the radio playing softly out in the living room, that Peggy would not have quit – that she experienced loss and heartbreak and did not quit, that she went on to change the world. I remember feeling that I could not let my hero down.

She saved my life that night.

She never quits. She always finds a way. She is grace under fire. She is femininity and strength. She is a tower. She has found love, and found friends, and found her way, no matter what life has thrown at her. She has changed her world – and mine – for the better. And in her, through her, I saw that my life was *not* over just because I felt like I had lost everything. There is still a chance for me to do good and make a difference. I was – I *am* – more than just the woman on the pedestal. I am still here. I am still here, and it is *not* over. And if I can help even one person the way Peggy has helped me, has inspired me — has saved me — then everything I have been through will be worth it. I spent so long hearing people tell me, "You can't," I started *believing* "I can't."

But I can. I have. I will. I know my value – I *finally* know my value, thanks to Peggy Carter and what she has taught me.

Cap said it in the comics, and Peggy said it in the movies: when everyone tries to tell you something wrong is something right, when they tell you to move – when *the whole world* tells you to move, plant yourself like that tree, and tell them, "No, *you* move."

RAGMAN
"Ragman & Jewish-American Identity"
by Dustin Hausner

If I mention characters like Superman, Spiderman, and Harry Potter, you know who these characters are. These are popular characters to mainstream audiences. People dress up as these characters, quote them, identify with them... and all of them celebrate Christmas. If you look through most fictional characters in mainstream American culture you will find that many of them celebrate Christmas. Now if you celebrate Christmas as well, you probably feel a specific connection with these characters. These characters have the same values and beliefs as you do and therefore you can connect with them based on those common religious values. There is nothing wrong with that. But, if you don't celebrate Christmas because of your beliefs, or religion, then there is a disconnect.

I am a Jewish person, and proud of my Jewish heritage, and I wanted to have a connection to superheroes who had a similar heritage, set of beliefs, religion, and culture as I do. As I tried to find a character to identify with, I looked through comics particularly, and while there are Jewish heroes like The Thing, from the Fantastic Four, Shadowcat from the X-Men, and a few others, most of them don't seem to have a Jewish culture. Magneto from X-Men and Moon Knight grew up Jewish, but later on didn't really acknowledge it except for in their back story. It seemed like the search to find a character who fit the bill would be in vain, and then I discovered Ragman from DC Comics.

Ragman was introduced in *Origin of the Tatterdemalion*, which was published in September of 1976. The character was created by Joe Kubert and Robert Kanigher. Originally the character didn't identify with a religion, and the character's name was Rory Regan. It was believed at the time that the character was Irish, which was later confirmed by the original writers. The 1976 series only lasted five issues. In 1991 the character was reintroduced in an eight issue miniseries.

It was in this new miniseries that the character was specifically identified as Jewish. In the back of the first issue of this 1991 miniseries this new revelation is explained by DC Comics Editor Kevin Dooley, *"Leo Keil of Brookline, MA, commented in old #3's letter column, then named "Junk Mail": "Despite this non-Jewish name, Rory seems, to me at least to be the comics' first Jewish super-hero...I like the idea." E. Nelson Bridwell said. Mr. Kanigher had stated, "If Rory was meant to be Jewish, he'd have a Jewish name...Rory is of Irish decent." Of course, being Jewish is more than a name, and that's not what Mr. Kanigher meant, but in this present version of RAGMAN, Rory is definitely Jewish, his powers heavily rooted in the Kabbalah."* In the third issue published November 1991, titled *The Origins of The Ragman* the origin of the Ragman suit is reinvented in a way that connects to Jewish persecution, Jewish folklore, and world history. This origin and connection is later built up in even greater detail in a Ragman one-shot titled, *Ragman: Suit of Souls* in 2010.

This origin of the suit was primarily expressed by the following ideas: Throughout the history of the Jewish people, they have been persecuted all around the world. The Ragman suit is created out of response to what happened in the Ghettoes of Prague during the 1500s. At that time Jews were being persecuted because of something called the Blood Libel. The Blood Libel was the accusation that Jews used the blood of Christian children to make matzah for Passover. Rabbi Loew, in response to his people's persecution, created a creature made out of clay called The Golem. The Golem was a soulless creature that at first protected the Jews but over time was not manageable. Eventually The Golem was destroyed and the council of Rabbis decided to create a suit of rags that had mystical powers.

The reason the council decided that a suit would be better was so a human being could control the magic. The Ragman suit was created and over the centuries different people used the suit and its magical abilities. Rory, in *Ragman Suits of Souls*, explains that the suit gives the person wearing it special powers. *"Strength. Agility. Speed. Limited Flight. Resistance. Even Immunity to many ordinary weapons. And the primary function of the Ragman: The ability to capture the souls of evildoers. Making them one more square in this patchwork suit...My costume is made up of hundreds of evil souls. I can draw on their strength, their knowledge, and their talents. It's not as cruel as it sounds. By helping me help others, they can earn redemption. An afterlife of salvation, instead of the eternal damnation that was their destiny."*

During the time of The Holocaust Rory's father, Jerzy Reganiewicz was bestowed the Ragman suit. After Jerzy immigrated to America, he changed his last name to Regan in part to protect his family from Anti-Semitism. Rory Regan would grow up knowing nothing of the Ragman until, years later, gangsters killed his father. Rory would find the suit and become the Ragman. In the few issues in which he has appeared Ragman has often fought against gangsters or demons.

This origin story is interesting for a few reasons. First, the persecution of Jews in the Ghettos of Prague due to the myth Blood Libel is an actual

Ragman

historical event that took place. As is the story of Rabbi Loew. The Golem is a famous Jewish Folklore story. The Holocaust was of course a horrendous event in world history and in both the 1991 series and the 2010 one shot, we see Rory's father did fight the Nazis. Due to The Ragman's suit having a "weakness to fire" and the souls in the suit preventing Jerzy from continuing to fight, he was unable to stop the genocide of over 6 million Jews.

The title of this essay is *Ragman: Jewish-American Identity*. The reason I chose the title is not simply because I connect with Ragman because he is Jewish, it is also because I feel that Ragman himself is in many ways a symbol of Jewish-American identity. The Ragman suit's origin is a combination of important history, Jewish stories, real life persecution, and the need for self-preservation. Many different rags maintain the Ragman suit, each representing the wanting of power and the wanting of redemption. Jews in the United States, belong to many different sects, Humanistic, Reconstructionist, Reform, Conservative, Orthodox, and others. These sects are like patches which come together and are the Jewish people.

The person inside the suit, Rory Regan, is constantly questioning himself about whether what he is doing is right, how to keep the rags together, and how to be good in so much darkness. Similarly, the Jewish American identity is all about the fundamental questions and principles that the Ragman Suit and Rory represent. The Jewish people have, in their long history, dealt with persecution, done their best to self-preserve, and now as in the past, questioned themselves about the right path in life, and being true to their heritage and culture while dealing with their personal values, and the world in which they live.

Ragman is not just a Jewish Superhero; he is the Jewish Superhero who represents me and the many different Jewish Americans. That is "why I geek" for Ragman, and why I will continue to promote him until the day he gets the recognition he deserves.

BOB DYLAN
"It's Delicate & Seems Like a Mirror"
by Will Dockery

> *"A [story] should have a beginning a middle and an ending... but not necessarily in that order." -Jean-Luc Godard*

I've told this story before, maybe more than once, but back in late 1973, the Bradley Memorial Library here in Columbus, Georgia had just two items on their shelves for folks wanting to encounter the work of Bob Dylan: *Tarantula* and *Self Portrait*.

That was it, nothing else.

Not the protesting folksinger, nor the thin wild electric nomad, nor even the simple country husband. No "The Times They Are a-Changin'", "Like a Rolling Stone", or "All Along the Watchtower". No, the budding Dylan acolyte in Columbus had to pick up either *Tarantula*, the free-verse novel entirely composed of stream of consciousness word etchings, or Self Portrait, the Dylan double album made up of an entirely personalized collection of covers and seemingly random outtakes of songs, which is still nearly universally critically panned.

How many people out there actually like *Tarantula*? How many have even read the darn thing? I have, many times, and love it madly. I love the wild mind of Dylan... the playful Trickster. The cutting bite words springing from the poison headache.

> *"The Censor in a twelve-wheel drive, semi-stopping in for donuts & pinching the waitress*
> *He likes his women raw & with syrup*
> *He has his mind set on becoming a famous soldier"*
> -Bob Dylan, *Tarantula*

Basically it is that old adage "Where were you when you first connected with the artistry of Bob Dylan?" and these were my formative texts, the huge influence *Self Portrait* and *Tarantula* have had on my own art... bizarre, yes, and that may explain /me/.

But... *Self Portrait* and *Tarantula*. Imagine if those were the only works of Dylan you'd ever experienced or ever would. And arguably either is enough to drive away newbies that were curious about what all the "fuss was about" on Dylan.

There was a cool feeling of "the present" in 1973-74, as each moment is or appears to be. Everyone buys into this, mostly... that the moment we are in is the ultimate, what came before is the rock and nothing greater could possibly happen. This was true in 1974 most definitely with Dylan... his glory days were over, conventional wisdom said...*Blonde on Blonde* was "so long ago", but actually only 7-8 years. It takes 7-8 years just to get up and get dressed nowadays, it seems, time moves so fast. But just 3 years after *Blonde On Blonde,* Dylan was already in his Country Western mode and the roaring electric rock was far away. It turns out that there were a thousand Dylans still ahead, Blood on the Tracks, Desire, the Christian phase, Infidels, the return to folk roots, Time out of Mind, the Christmas album, Chronicles, and old school Sinatra covers. But in 1974 the thought was that the end of the story had come, and I was just beginning mine.

It was in my granddaddy's barn in LaGrange, Georgia during the summer of 1969 when I first heard a Dylan song, "Lay Lady Lay", which was pleasant enough, but for a first listen... it could not compete with The Beatles that summer. The Beatles simply owned the summer of 69 for me and my cousin Jenny. Bear in mind that summer of 1969 was also when my own creations, the *Splut* and *Assemblers* stories, were coming out in episodes by the dozens... And I wrote and drew a vast majority of those in my granddaddy's chain saw shop. The first few *Splut* strips were created there, using my granddaddy's Poulan Chain Saw stationary. Good Lord how I miss La Grange... what a fool such as I to lose all that for ANY excuse. But, I digress...

> *"Ma Rainey & Beethoven once unwrapped a bedroll, tuba players now rehearse around the flagpole as the National Guard at a profit sells roadmaps for the soul..."*
> -Bob Dylan, "Tombstone Blues"

I was reading in Time and Newsweek about just how important Bob Dylan was, who, to me, had his biggest hit with "Lay Lady Lay" and now I listen to his 1970 double album to "Blue Moon" and the country style *Nashville Skyline* (which I had not heard yet, just the one single from it) style "Like A Rolling Stone". While reading Dylan's book *Tarantula*, his "novel", which was incredible almost gibberish, nonsense verse that made me think of John Lennon's prose.

One point to remember is that all this was happening in the space of just a couple of days, this very early perspective of Bob Dylan, but we all know how first impressions can stick, deep in the back of the mind... within a day or two I had Dylan's famous *Greatest Hits* volume and quickly flashed forward to the understanding of Dylan, the standard myth, young genius folk singer-protest songwriter, who went surreal and electric and changed the world, then got hurt and went away, until now... late 1973 when all the flurry of news was out on his grand return with the Band. I didn't actually buy an album of his on the day of release until *Blood on the Tracks*, which I found myself doing all the way up to *Empire Burlesque*. I don't know, maybe I ran out chasing *World Gone Wrong* down, also but I can't even seem to remember that year for some reason.

I can't realistically cover the entire 44 years I have followed Dylan intensely, so I just deal with the opening moments... 1978 would need at least a chapter, or a Russian novel to convey all that year, which also includes my firstborn son Clay's Origin Story. Empire Burlesque would make a funny, weird, sad, chapter. 1985... that black summer. It goes on, and there will be other chapters or whatever to detail those moments, if the Fates allow.

And yet my mind keeps returning to those first few days, before the wider world was opened to me, when I had just the two long form pieces of art, each weaving their way into my mind and embedding themselves in my psyche.

I think I may need to give a very short explanation of what *Tarantula* and *Self Portrait* are...they are not the most well know Dylan works, or not in most circles. Then again, look into them, find out for yourself... if you are unfamiliar, get set to have Bob Dylan blow your mind out and blow it back in again. For *Tarantula*, just like a comic book or television show might give a quick casual tag for an explanation... "Dylan's first book, a surreal cut-up affair..."

It is the same with *Self Portrait* ... there is no way I could describe that one in one sentence and convey the vast amount of contradictory and controversial history behind the album. What was once easily accepted as either the worst, or at the very least one of the worst, Dylan albums has now become known as yet another brilliant move, an exploration of thoughts and sounds that no one else had thought or dared to explore. It is that sense of daring that defines the artist to me, not the poetry or "voice of a generation" accolades, Dylan might be that, or might not. The interests to me are best found digging deep within the margins. I came upon the album, as the chapter states, without all that vast negativity, but it did make me wonder what all the fuss was about... it wasn't that the album was bad, but it certainly wasn't going to change the world. And yet I listened, and kept listening, and read the book, again and again. Lost in a spiral of poetic spider daydreams.

I had even read one short review of *Nashville Skyline* before I heard "Lay Lady Lay", some number of days or weeks before hearing it, and was very perplexed at the sarcastic tone of the writer, who said Dylan was now "fat and sassy", definitely not a compliment. That short review stuck in my head... and is still there, obviously.

This was the only Library in town back in those days and very popular with young folks of the day, really young folks from grade school to high school age, and who knows how many have that weird image Dylan projected on these works as their formative opinion of him...

Even now, I often daydream of Tarantula being made into a film on the order of say, "Yellow Submarine". I also see myself, in my youth, kicked back, visualizing the mad goings on... it is one hell of a book. Dylan has a way of expressing the world in pictures, which can be a truly transformative experience.

> *Thinking in pictures is...only a very incomplete form of becoming conscious. In some way, too, it stands nearer to unconscious processes than does thinking in words, and it is unquestionably older than the latter both ontogenetically and phylogenetically.*
> -- Sigmund Freud

The years passed in time, and more works became a part of my life. People met to have discussions and groupings and arguments and fights. I wrote and drew and created, from *Splut* on to *Demon House* and far beyond. For me, my own poetry became songs, performances and thoughts bleed together into a new way of thinking. Like the call of the novel finding its way into the corners of my life, through unknown avenues. And somewhere near the root, is Dylan, winding and weaving, an electric, terrifying, dreamscape inside a well worn, comforting, tune.

"One Hell of a poet, and lots of other things..." -Johnny Cash

Problems At Salisbury Fair
Playing a gambit
but still playing it straight.
Sent a fluff-girl downstairs
shaking her pompadour.

Silver badged shadow
boxing lady cop,
she carries a gun.
She sits at the piano with a
song
tight as a nun.

Clicking her flashlight
working old mimeograph.
We face our reflections
in the city of fishbowls.

Smoking with a journalist
over by the window.
Drinking strange mead
hesitates on delivery.

Working underground
flimflamming in the fog.
Picking minds
for breakfast couplets.

Bob Dylan

Shakes her Dickinson hair
Strolling by Salisbury Fair.

Crabbed picture reflects
as she inspects herself.
Winter is rugged
on the frail apple-tree.

Wrinkled man in a snow
cap
hip shaking
through Spanish Moss.

She quietly turns and runs,
from a silly basement bar.
Too much fun,
it was mostly a waste.

Helped her stagger to her
trailer
after drinking beer and
sniffing paste.
Some of this and a lot of
that
she shakes her tits with
tats.

Grinning from the stage
with her over sized
dentures.
Clicked her door to the
night
shutting out new
adventures.
Tight lipped little loser
stapling his chapbooks.

Shakes her Dickinson hair
Strolling by Salisbury Fair.

Will Dockery

Clicked his flashlight
asked was it him or them.
Saw the bloody handprint
no flat-lander
expectations.

One gone before she was
born
the other never born at all
they only exist because
she remembers them.

He's wound tight
by she who intoxicates.
The stone bag empty,
Sampson follows the
thunder.

Press her hands back
she's flat on her back
again.
Kiss the space
her face is open wide.

Stars sparkle bittersweet,
dripping from
these bearded lips.

Boss burbled
gobbledegook
chewing treacled tobaco.
He feeds on her mind like
a vulture
as she cries out jargon.

Shakes her Dickinson hair
Strolling by Salisbury Fair

- Will Dockery

114

THE X-FILES
"My Secret Agent Girl"
by Emma Caywood

> *Wasted away again in Scullyritaville,*
> *Searching for my lost piece of the plot.*
> *Some people claim that Agent Mulder's to blame,*
> *And I know*
> *It's partly his fault.*
> *But some people claim that Chris Carter's to blame.*
> *Now I know*
> *It's *his* bleepin' fault!*
> -Scullyritaville, by Sister Squat

I was 18 years old and a college freshman when *The X-Files* completely jumped the shark. It was the week of Valentine's Day in the year 2000. After 6.5 years of wondering what happened to Mulder's sister Samantha, we learned the truth. Was she kidnapped or murdered as part of a large government conspiracy? No. Was she abducted by aliens? No. Was she at least sucked up by the Flukeman? No. She was turned into starlight by the star people who come to humanely dissipate children before they are molested by the drunk Santa Claus at an amusement park. I guess. I only watched it once.

But that moment, the moment that I learned that everything to do with Chris Carter's plan for Mulder was complete crap, was the exact moment my life in Scully began.

But we're going to have to back up several steps, to a point before 18 year old me gets into a car with people she met over the internet (back when that was considered strange and scary) to drive 31 hours straight to Los

Angeles to see the actress who plays Scully do a monologue about the transcendent experience of looking at her vagina with a mirror.

One thing that is essential to following this chapter is understanding that it simultaneously has everything to do with Scully and absolutely nothing to do with Scully. Because... think of your very best friend. Perhaps you met them in math class, or in a sports ball league, or in your college Frat. But that's just how you met. You do many other things together now that do not involve mathematical formulas, aiming balls at a geometric shape, or drinking until you black out. Scully was just the beginning. What I mean to say is that Scully, as are The X-Files themselves, is the beginning and source of all things, but is not the only thing.

Scully: *Please explain to me the scientific nature of the "whammy"?*

Why *The X-Files*, though? Why anything? I can give you a long drawn out history of how my love for *Star Wars*, especially Princess Leia, brought me to science fiction, so I was primed to love a show written by all men with a kickass female secondary protagonist who was superior to all the men around her, but never got the respect she deserved. But fundamentally I fell in love with it the same way any preteen falls in love with any media property: it pinged something in my lizard brain that made me want to see more of it.

The mid 90s brought us *Xena*, but that level of camp didn't interest me, and brought us *Star Trek: Voyager*, but as much as I did watch it when it was on, *Star Trek* has always had too much standing around and talking for my liking. I had a love for *Northern Exposure*, especially the episodes with a fantasy, but Maggie and Shelley weren't exactly the best role models.

The X-Files

Scully was different. She was smart, she was as socially awkward as I was at that age, but she exuded a self confidence that I felt inside of myself, at least when I wasn't being expected to socially interact with my peers. I didn't think I was going to be a scientist, even though in middle school I was bussed to the high school for math classes and I took two AP science courses in high school, and I knew I wasn't planning on being in law enforcement of any sort. I wasn't Catholic (or religious), and my family wasn't military. I did have two brothers and a wild child female friend who lived with my family at the end of high school, but that might be the only similarity between my life and Scully's. But I knew her. I understood her in a way that I didn't usually understand anyone, fictional or otherwise.

But why *The X-Files*? For all that I am good with words, it's always been hard to explain what fandoms make my heart go pitter patter and what ones leave me cold. I like my science fiction to have nice banter-y dialogue. I like to laugh at shows that aren't primarily about being funny. The shows that I have been "all in" on are *The X-Files, Farscape, Buffy/Angel, Veronica Mars, Doctor Who/Torchwood, and The Walking Dead*. But I did spend a lot of my 20s prepping for and recovering from, surgeries, so there aren't a lot of shows that came out before 2007 that I haven't seen every episode of. Five disk at a time Netflix plans were a pre-streaming service perpetual patient's best friend. So I've had a chance to throw all in for a lot of different shows.

It's like falling in love. Sometimes my husband asks me why I married him. I always tell him that it's because he's funny and being with him was just as easy as being alone. (Coming from an introvert, that's high praise indeed.) But that's a terrible reason to have married someone. I find myself just as terrible at explaining why I spent the late 90s and early 00s "married" to the

X-Files or why I've "married" *Doctor Who*. There's something about those shows that makes my heart go pitter patter. There's something about sitting down for a new episode that makes my heart swell up. There's something comforting, but also exciting, about falling into those fictional worlds. They make me get a stupid smile on my face. I've been friends with a lot of television shows. I've even taken a few to bed with me. But I marry very few of them.

I started watching *The X-Files* in 1993, which was seventh grade for me. I loved the flashlights, the spooky stories, the mistrusting of the government, and the sexual tension (my mother had raised me on *Moonlighting*, and I knew good unresolved sexual tension when I saw it.) In high school, I discovered the world of fanfic, dirty and otherwise. I have a distinct memory of sitting in my attic room in high school and dialing up on the modem on my ancient C prompt – using IBM to pull up a handful of stories before I signed off the modem so no one would yell at me for being on it, and then reading the stories at my leisure. I remember watching the credits until the very last moment on FX reruns to get the season and episode number that flashed on the screen at the end (1X03 and the like) and then having to look at a master list of episodes so I could memorize episode names as I obsessively rewatched episodes. The children of today have it far too easy, I say with full understanding that at least I had cable reruns, VHS tapes, a VCR+, and alt.tv.x-files to help me gather information, unlike the true dark ages that came before me. But I did have to work for it. We didn't have gifs. We barely had screen caps.

There was a time when I could name an episode title from a still. There was a time when I could name an episode from a picture of Scully's outfit.

And this isn't *Doctor Who* where the costumes are usually distinctive: they were mostly skirt suits and I could tell them apart. We didn't cosplay, then, though. Cosplay was for *Star Trek* and Anime back then. I don't watch much *X-Files* now. I only have seen each episode of the new season twice. (Once as it aired, and the second time at a viewing party a friend hosted the next night. I keep making new Scully friends!)

But, and I know this happens to me with *Doctor Who* as well, when it's off the air, it becomes my nostalgia, my happy place. I forget about the ability for new episodes to get my blood pumping. But then I hear the wailing of the theme song and it's off to the races. But there's no science behind it. Not even that Scully could figure out.

Moulder: *Hey Scully, do you believe in an afterlife?*
Scully: *I'd settle for a life in this one.*

When I got to Northwestern, I bought an "I Want To Believe" poster that was taller than me for my dorm wall and this attracted a Sophomore that lived upstairs. She was the one who pushed me to join OBSSE, The Order of the Blessed Saint Scully the Enigmatic, a tongue in cheek order of "nuns" who were dedicated to Saint Scully, her Earthly Incarnation (Gillian Anderson), and her Plastic Incarnation (the Scully action figure.) It was basically a silly group of mostly overeducated women who thought Scully was very cool. It had a mailing list that, I soon found out, took 4 hours to get through on a post-show morning. I arranged my class schedule around it, since I found much of the episode conversation more stimulating than my peers' opinions on things in my freshman college courses, and I didn't want to miss my chance to engage with the conversation.

We'd also gather for the episodes on Sunday nights. I had watched new episodes with a handful of people when I was a teen, namely my high school boyfriend's parents and my camp friend Bethany I visited during spring break of my senior year, but mostly watching episodes involved me, alone, with the basement TV and all the lights off. Watching together with a no talking except during commercials policy brought me into the idea that television could be a group activity.

So, on to February 13, 2000. I had let my professors know that I would be missing that week's classes and that after that week's episode finished airing at 9 PM, I was going to drive from Chicago to Los Angeles straight through with two other women I'd met over the internet, so we could see Gillian Anderson give the mirror monologue in a celebrity studded cast of *The Vagina Monologues*.

It takes exactly 31 hours to drive straight from Chicago to Los Angeles if you basically never stop. And two 18 year olds and one 28 year old in a blue car named Sherman, with four PIs (Plastic Incarnations) of Scully riding on the dashboard can get to Los Angeles, delirious and giddy, and not even fully process the fact that the show itself had disassembled its own mythology 31 hours ago. Not to mention that the 28 year old had sprung for the front section tickets without telling us, and we were going to be able to go to the after party: my first Hollywood party.

The week was a blur of days taking pictures of our Scully action figures with alien looking seaweed on the beach, meeting up with other online friends of friends, drinking far too much, and all of my co-conspirators perhaps leaning into our obsessions a little too hard. The play was amazing. It was really during the peak of the popularity of that show, and the costumes were black dresses with red feather boas. I bought a red feather boa on Venice Beach before we left town. Before the show, we went down to the second row to ask Connie, Gillian's manager, if she would for certain be at the after party, since if she wouldn't, we wanted her to give Gillian the flowers we bought her. Gillian attended all the awards shows with her manager as her date, so she was easy to recognize. Connie said she'd be at the party.

She wasn't. That night I learned a very important thing that applied to every Hollywood party I would later attend when I worked as a literary manager for screenwriters: unless you are the honored guest, Hollywood parties generally have great food, terrible drinks, involve a lot of awkward standing around pretending you're not listening in on the conversations of people much more famous than you will ever be, and getting up the nerve to network with people who don't want to talk to you.

I still have never met Gillian Anderson. I have, however, met her mother, when the group of us volunteered for her charity, NF, Inc. She's very nice. I assume Gillian must be as well.

But, as I've said, it wasn't about Gillian.

Scully: *I have never met anyone so passionate and dedicated to a belief as you. It's so intense that sometimes it's blinding.*

That week was the first time I'd ever met more than a small handful of people I only knew from the internet. I knew the small Chicago crew of 5 other people, but before college, I'd never actually met my internet friends. In fact, most of my mailing list friends within my first fandom, Joni Mitchell, assumed I was a grown adult until I got over excited about getting my driver's license when I turned 16, and felt the need to brag on list, blowing the minds of people who had been my list friends for about two years at that point. (On the 90s internet, no one knows you're a teen.)

OBSSE Fest, Scully Summer Camp for Mean Adults happened for 4 days every summer. It was more of an anti-con than a convention. No panels, no special guests of any kind, but instead, a group of just over 100 Scully geeks taking over an off season resort in the summer. We had guitar sing-alongs in front of the campfire, a talent show, and the presentation of the cheeses (it's sort of what it sounds like, except it also involves foam cheese-heads and prom dresses.) I was in a cheerleader routine where we filked the opening scene from *Bring It On* about Scully, I performed a live interpretation of bad fanfic, and one year I co-hosted, dressed as a Bee. But mostly we just hung out, drank if we were of age, swam in the pool, played mini-golf, some people hooked up, and one year a bunch of us got tattoos. Some of us were gay, some bi, some SWILS (Straight Women in Love with Scully), and a handful were men. It was our chance to put names to the pseudonyms, and faces to the names.

That summer I arrived with the Chicago crew, and I left having been adopted into the just formed Hut of Evil, an extensive group of very funny and smart individuals, most of who had amused me with their posts in the past year. We created our own chat room, eventually our own mailing list, friended each other on live journal, and eventually on Facebook.

Remember, this was before being geeky was cool. This was before a high fantasy TV show about dragons and thrones and swords became normal Monday morning chatter among bros at the bro office. For a girl who grew up a bit lonely and a lot geeky, horribly bullied in middle school, was this meeting of like-minded internet people the first moment in my life where I felt socially competent, like I could come out of my shell and be the true me I was inside? Of course not.

Even if you ignore how cliquey it was, this is a group of people who grew up geeky somewhere between the 1960s and the 1990s. None of us was fundamentally well adjusted. My solace in a bunch of weird, queer, friendly, over-educated, mostly women did not lie in their kindness or acceptance. In fact, if I were to stumble upon a group with the level of dysfunction we had in that era now, I would run very quickly away. (We are currently a dysfunction free Facebook group.) But that was the thing about being a geek in the late 90s, early 2000s: we had all had a rough go of it before then. And the sort of bullying that went on resembled middle school, not the torture tactics and tumbling downward that goes on today. And most importantly, lists were closed circuits. Random people couldn't access and mock our conversations.

I didn't get involved with OBSSE for the friendships. I got involved because I found that my college coursework was missing something essential to the development of my mind. I needed a place where people over-analyzed things the same way I did, and the rough part about transitioning from a top high school to being a freshman in college is that liberal arts courses in college are significantly less demanding of both your brain and your time. Going from only getting 5 hours of sleep a night and a full schedule of school plus afterschool activities to a college schedule left me craving something that would give me more. And the thing about mailing lists is that they demand your attention in a way that any newsfeed cannot possibly demand. They fill your inbox, so choosing not to read a thread is a choice.

And this was before threads were combined, so you couldn't just skim past messages.

But then I found the friendships. I'm not in touch with any of the women I went to LA with, and I am still in touch with only one of the Chicago OBSSE women. But three people (+4 of their kids) at my wedding last summer were people I met on-list. And a lot of my friends can be parsed in degrees from OBSSE folk. (I met this person through this person who introduced me to this person...) There's a joke that when people ask you how your met someone from the list, some people say that we were in a book club, since "tongue in cheek pretend internet cult/nunnery devoted to the worship of Scully from The X-Files" tends to confuse people when you give that answer. Though it's actually much more amusing to be honest.

These days when you say you met someone over the internet, no one blinks an eye. My wedding also included a friend I met through a dating site, and the groom was someone I met at a Doctor Who convention. But people were afraid of meeting people over the internet in the late 90s/early 2000s. It just wasn't done. People over the internet were scary. Though I think I speak for all young geeks from the time before being a geek was cool when I say that people you meet at your school are scary. People over the internet are awesome.

Scully: *Sure, fine, whatever.*

The X-Files was a flawed show. And I don't mean it was flawed in the modern sense, though the rumor is that they did have in Gillian's contract for the first few seasons that she walk a few paces behind Mulder in walking shots. It was the 90s. That was par for the course. No, I mean that it was a giant conspiracy show where the writers didn't have a show bible.

Sometimes that revealed itself in confusing ways, like when Mulder forgot he was a psychologist in "Terms of Endearment", or when Scully says that they'll name their child William after his father, despite the fact that he hated his father, and she loved her father, who was also named William, or when Scully somehow managed to be pregnant for roughly the same length of time as a horse because, as Chris Carter points out, "they skip the summers."

But it mattered that they didn't know where they were going. One could argue that *The X-Files'* popularity despite clearly not having a plan for the central mystery of the show gave permission to shows like *Fringe* and *Lost* to create a show with a crazy mystery that they hope they will figure out later, thus ruining television forever. I know how television gets made. I do. Episodes are written with too little time and details are figured out as writers go along. But the central mystery needs to be laid out ahead of time, if only so that the writers know when to drop in subtle clues.

Had its mythology actually meant anything in the first place though? It was what hooked the plot together, what forced the writers to create and stick with character development. It prevented the show from being the sci fi version of *NCIS*. But when I think of the important character development I think of the episodes where Scully's father dies ("Beyond the Sea"), and where Scully finds out she might not die ("Clyde Bruckman's Final Repose"), and where she and Mulder get together ("all things?" Sort of?) I don't think about black oil or code talkers or little grey aliens or the Cigarette Smoking Man. I think of the moments inserted into what were essentially Monster of the Week episodes. I think about the mytharc beyond the mytharc, the proto-Buffy format of just having your Big Bad plot happen during the monster of the week episodes.

That being said, Mulder's main thrust, his whole reason for pursuing The X-Files in the first place, was his need to discover what happened to Samantha. And the writers failed that. It's almost as if they didn't know where the show was going when they planned the show in the first place.

Scully: *What if there was only one choice and all the other ones were wrong? And there were signs along the way to pay attention to.*

At the end of our Los Angeles week, 6 AM that Saturday, as we were heading back northeast to connect up with 40 east, I was the only person awake when I drove Sherman over a giant piece of tarp. It had flown off the back of a pickup, and there was no avoiding it. But I looked in my rearview, and there was the tarp. So I didn't wake anyone up about it.

But as I kept driving, I started hearing the sort of kerthump of an old broken highway, the sort of rhythmic kerthump that you often hear in places where roads break down with weather: the only sorts of places I'd lived in. So I turned up the mixtape we'd made of songs that made us think of Scully, and kept driving.

It was only when people started waking up and wanting coffee that they pointed out that the kerthumping had gotten louder. So we pulled over at the next service station, which sent us to a service station down the road. We went off on foot, in the middle of the desert by this point, and they looked into the kerthump.

The X-Files

When we got back, they told us that there was a whole mess of tarp that had ripped off from the bigger tarp wound up in the wheelbase of the drivers' side front tire. And that if we'd kept going, the car might have ended up exploding.

Reading this will be the first time my mother hears about this near death experience, so I hope the metaphor I'm working toward holds up. The tarp is the starlight. We drove over it, it got caught up in our wheelbase, and it probably should have exploded us. But it didn't. We kept watching. Or we didn't.

I've actually never seen the Episode "William". I was doing something else on April 28, in the spring of my Junior year of college, and my VHS didn't properly record. And then I read the list traffic the next day, about buffalo mobiles and Scully being willing to give away her second child, after the first was snatched from her, and after being told she was infertile. I gathered it was something about protecting him from the government/aliens/I don't know, maybe starlight, too. I liked to brag that since I hadn't seen it, I had plausible deniability, and therefore it might not have happened. All my list mates supported my decision. I wish I had missed that one where Kathy Griffin played her own twin, too. It would be nice to deny that one happened as well.

But the point is that we kept going. We got into other fandoms together. Many of us still vacation together. I'm in a secret Facebook politics group started by a member, I'm friends with people's kids, and a few women in the group left their husbands for each other. (They became more than just SWILS.) We all have Scully to thank for that. Or maybe Gillian. Sadly, probably Chris Carter as well, though the last great thing he did for the show was fight

127

for Gillian to get the role. We have the internet to thank. Or maybe just each other.

> *Because it's not just about Scully. But it's a little about her.*
> *Oh my Scully, Agent Scully, your monotone turns me on.*
> *You can do an autopsy while firing your gun.*
> *Your hair and makeup looks great, even while you're saving the world.*
> *Mulder gets killed at least once ev'ry year, and it's getting so old that*
> *we really don't care, but our Scully she's always alive and she's well, and*
> *I know that someday she'll be my Secret Agent Girl.*
>
> -Eric D. Snider

STAND-UP COMEDY
"From Convention Halls to Brick Walls: How Geeks Got Me to Stand Up"
by Hannah Harkness

When I tell people I'm a stand-up comedian, I get two responses more than anything else. The first is "Ooh, tell me a joke!" aka, "Dance, puppet!" That one I usually respond to by telling someone it's awkward to do in that context, or a begrudging one liner if they won't leave me alone. The second is "where do you do comedy?" I like answering this one, because I get to look people in the eye and say "Doctor Who Conventions".

These days I actually perform at comedy clubs, bar shows and theaters, but I grew my roots making reference-heavy inside baseball jokes at cons. When I first started doing comedy when I was 19, I was riddled with irrational outsider anxiety that prevented me from interacting with the comedy community at all. I was a huge stand-up nerd. I could recite Eddie Izzard DVDs start to finish, I loved George Carlin, and my friends and I would crack each other up quoting Margaret Cho all the time. But I was a little Goth anime nerd that spent most weekends crashed on tiny floor spaces in convention room hotels.

I started volunteering and working at comic book conventions when I was 17 and it was most of my world socially until my early 20s. Nerd culture made me who I was, but it was a bubble. There were zero nerd girls on Comedy Central. Honestly, there weren't that many women at all, and many of the ones that did exist looked like women that would have bullied me in in high school. The idea of going to a comedy open mic filled with mostly older single men and only one or two women with whom I had nothing in

129

common was not only daunting socially, it was also more or less impossible because everything was in bars and I wasn't old enough to drink.

The year after I graduated high school was a strange and formative one for me. Despite loud protests from my guidance counselors, I didn't immediately go to college. I had originally planned to go to art school, but after going to a few daunting portfolio reviews and hearing cautionary tales about job prospects on the other side, I got cold feet and decided to join City Year. City Year is a branch of Americorps that gives you a stipend and partners you with a group of people to do immersive community service for a year. It was rewarding and life changing and I received a scholarship large enough to get me through my first semester of college, but it was hard work. I had to wear a strict uniform and work long days in a dangerous neighborhood. On certain days I did physical labor like repainting fences, planting trees, or even trash removal from a local reservoir. Then I'd go home at night to my parents' house. I'd look at social media and see all of my friends who had moved away from home partying it up at college. It was a hard year and I frequently felt depressed and left out. All of my friends were gone, I was overworked and underpaid and I needed somewhere to go.

One day when I was walking around my neighborhood, I saw a sign on the door of a newly opened hookah lounge for a Wednesday night open-mic which would have comedy, music, and poetry. Unlike the bars where most open-mic nights or stand-up acts are held, you only had to be 18 or older to go to the hookah bar. I decided that I would finally try stand-up comedy, maybe there really wouldn't be any other convention nerds there, but because it was a music and poetry open mic too, there would at least be other women that were cool and artsy. I hastily typed a set on my parent's computer. I wish I could remember it – it was very Eddie Izzard inspired absurdist stuff, not anything like what I do now. Nervous as hell, I memorized my lines and signed up the following Wednesday.

Thankfully, I did well. There were no comedians at this mic that would have told me that everyone bombs at first – if I had bombed that might I might have never tried again. I left that night walking on air and suddenly having made a whole room of new friends, and feeling cool as hell because a lot of them were musicians a few years older than me. As I left, one of the women who ran the open mic, Liza, came up to me and held both of my hands and said, "Come back and bring the funny with you". After that, I never missed a Wednesday. I didn't always do well, but at that point the regulars knew I was funny and that was the only thing that mattered to me.

But like all writers, I wanted to write what I knew, and most of what I knew was nerd culture. I did my first set that was about conventions and involved nerd references one Wednesday. As a gag I had Liza hold up subtitle cards explaining what the hell I was talking about when I made a reference that she would change whenever I clapped twice. It crushed, but I knew in my head that what I really wanted to do was make nerd references to a crowd that would immediately understand what I was talking about. I thought that was impossible, so I didn't really consider trying to find a place to take that kind of act.

Eventually I finished City Year and went to college. Comedy more or less went on hiatus at that point. I did one or two shows but I was mostly too busy with conventions, school, and extracurricular activities to really pursue comedy at all. College was my convention heyday – I went to San Diego comic con four times. I interned with a few publishers, volunteered, and even sold corsets at one point – whatever I needed to do to get a badge, I was on it. I did comedy at one or two random variety shows, but that was it. At one point, I miraculously won a talent show held by the Greek organizations on campus, which resulted in drunk frat dudes yelling "Yo, it's that funny chick!" from the porches of frat houses for the rest of my college career. My favorite was when a guy in salmon shorts and a backwards baseball hat stumbled up to me on the street at 2am while I was wearing full Goth regalia. I was preparing for him to make fun of me, but instead he said "Yo, you're that funny chick, right? You should make a profile, I'd totally read it!" We high fived and then he stumbled off into the night, probably to vomit or publicly urinate.

I first tried stand up in the actual comedy scene the year after college, but I didn't go back with any real consistency. I only went to maybe three or five open-mics tops, and during them I had difficulty making friends. One day, I bombed hard for the first time in my life. With nobody to tell me that happens to every comic, I was too humiliated to go back. I had also slipped into a pretty deep post-college depression. Once again I was separated from my friends. I had a women's studies degree and I had gotten cold feet on going immediately to graduate school to continue studying in that field. I was working a dry receptionist job and just barely making rent.

One day, the talent booker for a convention I went to a lot, Wicked Faire, called me. Wicked Faire was billed as an annual indoor winter renaissance faire, but it was a lot more than that. It had a lot of those elements, but it was mixed with miscellaneous geek culture, circus arts, and sex-positive workshops. But mostly, it was a PARTY. Most mornings I'd wake up on a hotel room floor covered in glitter with a pounding headache, wondering how much mead I had the night before or how many corseted women I had made out with. The talent booker said that he had heard I did stand-up comedy and wanted to know if I could do a set for an hour. Having mostly watched comedy specials on TV, I said yes, of course-I mean that's what comedians do, right? I had no idea at that point that most comics spend years crafting their first hour. Sometimes I still wonder how I didn't violently bomb that set.

But I realized, that this was IT. This was my time to write all the nerd reference heavy jokes that I had always wanted to write. Everyone there would understand my jokes and I would get to perform in front of all of my friends I had known for years. I got to writing. That 45 minute set is still up on my YouTube channel in pieces. While I can't really take most of that material to most of the gigs I currently get booked on, it was the material that really gave me confidence in my writing and made me think that I could be successful. I wrote about steam punk, Nintendo, cranky GameStop employees, Doctor Who, anime – whatever I wanted, for the first time. And I crushed on camera. After those two 45 minute sets, I walked out of the convention finally believing in myself. I wrote material that everyone could understand that I could take to normal comedy shows, walked into open mics knowing for sure that I was good. I made my first comedy friends and the rest was history.

More nerd opportunities came later on. The Rocky Horror Picture Show cast I have performed with for over a decade began letting me open for them. Nerd comedy showcases and podcasts found me and booked me. I produced a show at Broadway comedy club with nothing but comedians I had met on Brian Michael Bendis' message board. Then one day I got a call from the same guy who booked me on Wicked Faire. It was the first year of ReGeneration Who and he wanted to know if I could swing a half hour of Doctor Who jokes. I immediately said yes. With 50 years of source material about a time traveling alien in a phone booth, it honestly wasn't even that hard.

Over the three years ReGeneration Who has been running, I've had the opportunity to do my own show, host the main panel room, and perform on the zany and hilarious "Dave Ross Variety Hour" hosted by Terry Molloy. I even got to interview one of my heroes, Patricia Quinn – the original actress to play Magenta in the *Rocky Horror Picture Show*. ReGeneration Who is my favorite gig. Nowadays I'm slowly beginning to get booked on shows where I rub shoulders with people who have TV credits, but I'm still seen as a rookie – most comics are until they've been working the clubs for 10+ years or get a TV credit. But at ReGeneration Who, I feel like a star. I'm listed as a featured guest on the website alongside actors and actresses I've been watching since I was a kid and I get to share a green room with them. Attendees that have been there since the beginning remember me. I get complimented all weekend and my own hotel room. This is because of show-runner Oni Hartstein's commitment to treating all guests and performers equally, but I can't stress how much that means to a performer used to getting no pay to do comedy for five minutes in the backs of bars in Philadelphia.

I love many of the people I've met in the comedy scene, and I'm relocating to New York this year because there are some clubs like the Creek and the Cave in Queens that I've started to call a second home. But I'll never forget that the places I really cut my teeth and began to believe in myself were ballrooms with ugly carpets and harsh lighting where half the audience is dressed like robots. And if someday I make it big, you'll never hear me stop thanking geeks. And make no mistake, I'm going to keep doing ReGeneration Who – if that event is good enough for people who have played The Doctor, it will always be good enough for me.

SUPERNATURAL
"Supernatural, Naturally: A True Tale of a Moose, a Squirrel, & the Nut Who Loves Them"
by Dawn Ferchak

So, apparently, sometime in the fall of 2005, my sister, along with several of my friends, started telling me about this show I should watch. This show had two super-hot guys and it was all about chasing monsters and ghosts, and – "Get this," they said – "it's even called Supernatural." "They could have called the show *Shit Dawn Likes*," they said. "Now with extra hot guys and a muscle car. Go! Watch!"

At least, they claim they said this. I don't remember any of this. This doesn't sound like the kind of thing I would have ignored. It's got all the things I like. But if those friends are telling the truth, then I missed it. Somehow the show's existence fell off my radar and I never got around to it, and then other things happened and I forgot all about the two hot brothers and their muscle car. I'd hear the name sometimes, or see the merch, and briefly my brain would go, "Oh, yeah, the hot ghost-hunting brothers show. Gotta get on that." But by then Netflix was streaming and I had a million new shows to try to watch, along with the shows I was already watching. And there it went, off the radar again.

Then came 2013, when my life started to fall apart. I won't get into those details-- they don't matter. Basically, things started going down the shitter and I didn't want to believe it, and I needed something to watch while I hid in bed and pretended that everything was fine, thank you. I had struck up a new friendship recently, and she was a superfan of Supernatural, so I figured, "This is a good time for eye candy and things that don't exist." Then someone else told me that Jim Beaver, an actor of whom I was already a huge fan from his stellar work as Whitney Ellsworth in Deadwood (possibly my favorite show of all time), played Bobby Singer on Supernatural, and I finally started watching.

I'd love to say I got hooked right away. I might have, actually, but I don't really remember. You see, "started to fall apart" turned into "total fucking implosion." Things went from bad to worse, and your humble narrator checked herself into a nuthouse for a little while, followed by a six-month mental health leave from work.

A six-month leave from work means a lot of free time. Like, a LOT. Even with all the therapy appointments, there's still a lot of time where you've got nothing to do, to say nothing of the nights you're not really sleeping anyway. So it was roundabout late September or early October of 2013 when I renewed my acquaintance with the charming Winchester brothers and started watching the series from the beginning.

On October 14, 2013, I started my first Supernatural fanfic. I just checked the date in my google drive. So that didn't take long at all. Glory be and pass the shotgun shells, Supernatural claimed another one. Praise Chuck.

All those people who recommended I watch the show way back in 2005 were totally right, and I do kinda kick myself for not having jumped on this most excellent bandwagon a long time ago. But no matter—I have since thrown myself in wholeheartedly, and I don't regret a single thing.

Let's talk about the show itself, first: Supernatural hits all my buttons. Let's start with the base ones, shall we? It's escapism, pure and simple, like a lot of my favorite books, films, and television shows. It has stunningly attractive leads Jensen Ackles (Dean Winchester) and Jared Padalecki (Sam Winchester), to say nothing of all the rest of the male pulchritude eye candy upon which I happily feast my eyes: Jeffrey Dean Morgan (John Winchester), Misha Collins (Castiel), Mark Sheppard[1] (Crowley), Richard Speight, Jr. (Gabriel—my #1 SPN boyfriend), Rob Benedict (Chuck Shurley), and Matt Cohen (young John Winchester and the archangel Michael).

Gosh, that's a lot of men, isn't it? At its heart, SPN exists in a man's world, it's true. The show is about two brothers (and initially their father) in a world that is primarily male—hunters of the supernatural. There's been a hell of a lot of criticism about it, too. My opinion? Those people haven't paid enough attention, because the recurring female characters on SPN are amazing-- amazing enough that a few are getting their own show, Wayward Daughters. But from the beginning, there were solid, strong female characters, good girls and bad. On the good side, we had Missouri Moseley, Pamela Barnes, Ellen and Jo Harvelle (mother and daughter), Eileen Leahy, Sheriff Jody Mills, Sheriff Donna Hanscum, Alex Jones, Claire Novak (those four are the Wayward cast, so far), Linda Tran, Mary Winchester, and the amazing Charlie Bradbury (played by the incredible Felicia Day). You like it bad?? I've got your bad. Demons Ruby 1.0 and Ruby 2.0 (who is now married to Jared Padalecki in real life), and Meg 1.0 and 2.0. Demon queen Lilith. Knight of Hell Abbadon. Baddies but maybe kinda goodies? Sure -- Angels Naomi and Hannah, witch Rowena, and God's very own sister, Amara.

---

[1] Nerd Royalty, having been on the likes of The X-Files, Firefly, Battlestar Galactica (reboot), Doctor Who, Leverage, and more. If you don't know who this guy is, turn in the nerd card or work on upping your cred.

Reapers Billie and Tessa. Some came to good ends; some to bad. And a few got less than they deserved, including some outright fridging. Do I have issue with how some of these women were taken out? Damn right I do. But their deaths don't take away from their incredible characterizations and their BAMF power. And for the record? Most of them pass the Bechdel test. Stick that in your Devil's Trap and salt it.

Then there's the lore. Lots and lots and LOTS of lore. For someone who cut her teeth on mythology books and urban legends, this show is meaty and delicious. It has monsters and folklore and urban legends and ghosts (I am a horror girl from way back, so this pleases me no end.). In this show, research matters. Books matter. Knowledge matters. Can the pretty boys kick ass? Of course they can. But they can also go to a library (in the beginning) or google (more common now) and find shit out. Hunters have to know the lore or they die. In the world of Supernatural reading is more than just fundamental. The right book will literally save your life. Study hard and maybe you'll live.

Plus, there is a complex, overarching mythos that, when it's done well, is worthy of a place in the American mythic pantheon alongside shows like *The X-Files* (a big inspiration for SPN, which is particularly clear in the first two seasons). It's not always done well--look, I love my show, but everybody makes mistakes. There have been bad episodes; hell, there have been bad seasons. But somehow--at least so far--they manage to pull it out of the muck and get back on track. And when they are on, they are ON.

The best SPN episodes run the emotional gamut. When they make fun of themselves, in eps like "The French Mistake," "The Monster at the End of This Book," "Changing Channels," "The Real Ghostbusters," and the amazing musical episode, "Fan Fiction," it's glorious and very, very funny. When they hit the emotional buttons hard and fast, in episodes like "No Rest for the Wicked," "When the Levee Breaks," "Swan Song"[2], "Death's Door," and "Regarding Dean," it's gut-wrenching and ugly crying. Serious ugly crying.

But for my money, it's the eps that manage to combine the two that are my favorite. The moments in eps like that are golden, the way the writers can make your emotions turn on a dime--that's life, you know? One moment you're laughing, and the next, you get hit by a bus. Or someone you love does. In an unnatural world, Supernatural feels natural. Of course we care about these characters, ridiculous though they may be. How could we not? How could we not feel the terrible choices when the Trickster tries to show Sam what life without Dean will really be like and why that might have to happen, in "Mystery Spot"? How could we not weep when Dean and Sam finally have to let Bobby go, in "Survival of the Fittest", and each fleeting time after that when they caught glimpses of him? The best of the SPN writers play our fandom hearts like marionettes on a string, and we love it. We really do.

But wait, there's more. So much more. There's the fandom. The SPN fandom is an astonishing place. Of course we have our share of crazies, like all fandoms do. But this fandom—encouraged by the cast—wants to move mountains and tries to very often. Need to raise money for a charity? We're on it; just ask Misha Collins and Random Acts, or Jared Padalecki and Always Keep Fighting. There's a line from Season 3, Episode 16, where Bobby Singer says, "Family don't end with blood." Well, we took that line and we ran with it, and the cast joined right in. The stars and co-stars of SPN are deeply involved with charitable works and have started many of their own, such as

---

[2] Originally, the series was meant to end here. Horrifying, right? I KNOW!

Supernatural

Jared Padalecki's "Always Keep Fighting" campaign, born out of his own struggles with depression and mental illness. I have heard it more than once--Supernatural saves lives. With AKF and all that has grown out of it, it actually does.

At the conventions, there are tables manned with volunteer support staff for fans having mental health issues (within reason, of course, and professionals are definitely brought in when appropriate). Fans will spot someone having a rough time or a panic attack, and they will step in to talk, bring water, help calm, whatever is needed. Jared has been known to stop if he sees someone starting to panic (please DO NOT start faking panic attacks to get Jared's attention--don't be that fan). Hugs and gentle words abound from all the SPN cast members at photo shoots, even sometimes during Q&As. They walk the walk. It surprised the hell out of me, to be honest. But they walk the walk. It's amazing. But don't just trust my words. Here are some from (one of the) horse's mouth; this was part of Richard Speight, Jr.'s intro at the most recent Supernatural convention in Vancouver, Canada, on August 12, 2017:

> If you have never been in this room, if you have never come to a convention, if you've never watched a video of a convention, if you've never experienced the power of the fandom either online or in person, you do not understand what it is and how it works and how powerful it can be. It is a force to be reckoned with. It is a fandom like no other. It is not just a group of people who like a TV show and gather together to get pictures with people from that show. It is a force of people who do not care about your color, who do not care about your sexual preference, who do not care about who you are, what you do, who you

*love, how you love, why you love what you do and why you do it. They
care that you are good to yourself and good to others. And when you do
that, and they do that to you, and it becomes this giant chain of cool
people doing the right thing for the right reasons, THAT is the
Supernatural fandom.*

Have I mentioned that he's my favorite? Because he is totally my
favorite. But I digress. Did SPN save my life, personally? No, not really. But it
kinda saved my soul, because it gave me something to smile about when I
felt like I'd never smile again, and it gave me a whole new group of friends
when I really needed some, and it gave me something to focus on that wasn't
a great bloody mess. It went a long way to healing my heart. It still does.

It's easy to get overwhelmed by the idea of a fandom and also by a long-
running show. I have a few friends who flatly refuse to watch SPN on two
primary grounds: the fandom is full of the crazies and there are eleventy-
billion episodes. Since I covered the former above, let's hit the latter. Yes,
there is a lot to catch up on. Season 13 will start in the fall, and as far as
anyone knows right now, there might be more beyond that. This is not a
weekend binge-- there are 264 hours of show to get through, so far. That's
11 solid days. It's a commitment, I get it. Maybe you could skip forward a
little and start with, say… season… hang on, I am trying to find a good place
to just start watching…still looking…Balls, I can't find a place to just pick up
and begin. Because it all ties back, you see. Things get brought up from
seasons back, and suddenly they're important. So it's a commitment. But it's
worth it, I promise. I swear on Baby. And that's saying something.

PRO-WRESTLING
"Fake: Wrestling's F-Bomb"
by Alex Fitzgerald

"Fake." That is the dreaded word that every person in my fandom has heard at least five times on the playground during grade school. I say grade school, because once you hit an age, usually your mid-teens, you realize that bringing up this particular fandom isn't socially acceptable in the slightest. God forbid your best friend finds out you're a fan, or even worse, a girl you like hears that you are interested in "that fake nonsense". My chosen fandom, the one that I still love and watch and care about, Pro-Wrestling, is usually greeted with these statements and more.

When you are a Pro-Wrestling fan it means spending the rest of your school days until graduation being pelted with cries of, "You know it's fake!" or even off handed asides of, "They use blood packets." (Now, as for the blood packets, they actually do cut themselves in an act called "blading", which involves taking a razor or sharp object to your forehead and slicing it open, after safely taking a bump to the head. That part isn't really fake at all. Take that, grade school bully!) Now I admit, yes, most of those grade school insults are in fact true, and it is "fake". That being said, the fact that it is fake is (almost) completely irrelevant. What really defines the term "fake" and why is it considered the worst of all f-bombs to wrestling fans? More importantly, why stay a fan of something that gets such harsh backlash in everyday life?

For me personally it all started in 1999, which many consider the heyday of modern professional wrestling. There were three major organizations; the World Wrestling Federation (now known as World Wrestling Entertainment),

World Championship Wrestling, and Extreme Championship Wrestling, with the latter two going out of business in 2001. At that point in time, there were over twenty hours of wrestling available to watch over various cable networks on top of the merchandise flooding places like Target and Kmart. You had various different lines of action figures, with some that had talking microchips, some that had "neck snapping action" and even a set that made fake sweat. Wrestling was unavoidable, and it's not shocking that 1999 was the year that drew in the attention of the most new fans the sport would ever see, including five year old me.

The first professional wrestling show I ever watched was an episode of *WWF Smackdown!* Smackdown was designed and marketed as a PG show to counterbalance the TV-14 *Monday Night Raw*. While Raw aired from 9:00pm until 11:00pm on the USA network, Smackdown aired an hour earlier from 8:00pm to 10:00pm on UPN. In reality Smackdown was just as vulgar and raunchy as its sister show. The show followed the same storylines, just with some of the more colorful language censored and the bloodiest and most graphic scenes edited out as well. With that being said, it worked like a charm, and I was able to watch Smackdown every night before bedtime.

The first character that really grabbed my attention was a rotund masked man who went by the name "Mankind". Mankind was portrayed by Mick Foley, one of the best entertainers that wrestling has ever seen. He would stop at nothing to entertain a crowd, including putting his body on the line. A year prior, Mick was chucked off of a sixteen foot high cage, resulting in him suffering bruised ribs, a dislocated jaw, and a major concussion. Even after going through all of that, he still performed the next night. Now we have concussion safeguards and a better understanding of various medical situations that would have prevented his continued work but at that time it just served to make Mick Foley seem indestructible. Eventually his body began to slow down from the various injuries he sustained during his career, but to his credit, he had another ace up his sleeve which he played just around the time I began watching.

Mick, on top of being one of the most brutal and hardcore wrestlers ever, also had a comedic edge like no one else before him. As he began to wind down his career, he covered for the fact that his physical skills were no longer top notch by making everyone laugh in insane ways; from using a sock puppet to choke out opponents, to creating an entire *This Is Your Life* based event for The Rock's birthday (with Mick finding out he had the date wrong at the end); Mankind was able to become a loveable underdog that rallied everyone behind him. Set up from the goodwill he obtained from putting his body on the line for the entire audience and prolonged by his perfect comedic timing and sense of humor, Mankind became an intense draw for everyone. This included a five year old me, sucked in by the antics of this weird man in a leather mask talking about terms I didn't know the meaning of, such as "testicular fortitude".

While Mankind was the main character that drew me in, he also had a very strong supporting cast "on the program", so to speak. This being the late nineties and the first years of the new millennium, the WWF borrowed heavily from the pop-culture of the time with the other characters on the program seeming like they had jumped out of various famous shows of the era. You had an evil prison warden who would batter opponents with a nightstick, akin to an episode of *COPS*. There were vampires that spit a "red viscous liquid", since you couldn't have them drinking blood on a PG program that seemed to have jumped right out of an episode of *Buffy The Vampire Slayer*. There was even a pimp character, complete with bright outfits including airbrushed vests and pants, inspired by the rappers at the time. It was a melting pot of all these different pop culture tropes with larger than life performers playing them. They were almost like comic book characters.

Wrestling, of all things, was the gateway for me to get into comics. The big ones that hooked me in were the *Spider-Man* and *X-Men* cartoons that aired on weekend mornings on Fox Kids. *Batman: The Animated Series* and *The Incredible Hulk* had a lasting influence on me as well. Each show had larger than life heroes and villains battling it out for good and evil. Flashy characters, each with fleshed out backstories and relatable traits, embroiled in feuds with characters that were their mirrored opposites in many ways. There would even be crossovers where characters would team up to take on groups trying to tear down everything they stood for. Now the funny thing is – I was talking about wrestling the entire time there. The same ideas are used in both wrestling and superhero stories; the hero and villain tropes, extensive battles, and fighting over something they hold dear, be it morals or a title belt. Those similarities really got me into that genre of storytelling and I have wrestling to thank for that.

Much like comic books, where Marvel and DC have distinct styles, so too do the companies that produce the different Pro-Wrestling shows. My stepdad handed down some of his old tapes from an older wrestling promotion called the National Wrestling Alliance. At that point in time the tapes were around eighteen years old and were completely different from anything I had ever seen. Instead of the flashy characters, fast paced storyline, and even quicker pace and style I was used to, this classic wrestling

146

was slower with far more down to earth and simpler characters. You had Dusty Rhodes, a charismatic son of a plumber that fought for the common man. Ric Flair, a showboating egomaniac that always wore the newest in fashion and cheated at every turn. Nikita Koloff, your run of the mill evil Russian who assaulted enemies with chains. The match pacing was also much different, while a typical WWF match would be over in ten minutes, an NWA match could go on for upwards of an hour.

To put it in perspective, it's a lot like going from a bright *Avengers* film, to a brooding Christopher Nolan *Batman* flick. Both have the right amount of pacing and character development, but with one there's more comedy throughout, while the other has a bleaker outlook on the events. In both worlds the same theme of good versus evil is there, with good prevailing. For example, while WWF would have a world title feud involving celebrities with them helping the champion, the NWA would have the main good guy get his leg broken, have the title taken from him by the bad guy, and follow his rise to taking the belt back. Different styles, but they both have the same outcome.

Another important piece of this story is the timeline of what was happening with wrestling after I started watching. While I started at the height of wrestling's popularity there was a soon a steep decline in popularity. It went from a thing a kid was able to talk about actively on the playground with his friends in 2001 to an object of heavy ridicule in the same environment in 2004. The real reason for this change was unknown. With something that has been on as long as pro wrestling there are bound to be certain fluxes in viewership. One large reason could have been the stars retiring, which huge stars like "Stone Cold" Steve Austin and The Rock did in

2003. Network changes also came into play, with Raw moving from USA to TNN (now Spike) in 2001. Or perhaps it was just a change in style trends, much like how during the same time period, fewer and fewer people would wear fanny packs. So, all things considered, I had to really love it to stick around through a dark period, which I absolutely did and still do. It's also good thing I did.

To this day the best way to really talk about wrestling, and to find other fans, is online. Through forums and chatrooms people would gather to talk about the ins and outs of what was going on. It was a space that wouldn't make anyone feel awkward or dumb for being a fan of something that isn't a social norm. I'm happy to say I met most of my best friends this way. We started just talking about wrestling but soon moved on to other subjects like stand-up comedy and TV shows like The Simpsons, and then we progressed to actually giving one another advice and eventually to hanging out in person. It's odd that something like wrestling fandom could give me a form of family, but it absolutely did.

Through all of the stigmas and inabilities to connect with people firsthand over it, my love of wrestling stuck with me, for a variety of reasons. The first is the fact that these characters appear nearly every day of the week and nearly every week of the year in some capacity. That's nearly six to eight hours of televised content every single week. No other medium can really keep up that pace and stay fresh. Imagine if there was a new Marvel movie every month of the year, let alone every week? How sick of *The Walking Dead* would the populace be if there was a new episode every seven days like clockwork? It's hard to think about, but one of my main draws to wrestling is the fact that it is intense action for multiple hours every week that doesn't get repetitive. It's the Holy Grail of entertainment in my eyes, never becoming frail or slowing down.

The other big reason wrestling stuck with me is that it could be considered a "breathing entity". You can't visit an episode of *Game of Thrones*, but you can absolutely sit in on an episode of Raw. You can't really check in on what The Doctor is doing with your own eyes (unless you want to be arrested for stalking), but the character of someone like John Cena is much easier to check in on during what could be considered "everyday life". Can't make it to a TV event? Your favorite wrestlers are always on tour, so you can see live, un-filmed episodes of the show close to you, with the stories fitting in-between the main narrative. Plus, this universe does not present a danger to you personally, unless you're a wrestler. As fun as being in the same universe as Batman may be that means you're probably going to worry about a living Scarecrow gassing you to death on a daily basis.

Overall, professional wrestling opened my eyes to an entire genre of entertainment that just fit my personality like a glove. It provided me with real life superheroes without me even realizing it, all while opening the door to the superhero genre. I don't stay a fan of Pro-Wrestling out of a sense of loyalty either. It's something that I really do still heavily enjoy, with different flavors so to speak, that I can taste without end. It does help that it's a constant, with no off season, always going every week. It's a train ride I don't intend to hop off of any time soon. It's a linear program that I can pick up on anywhere at any time and be completely comfortable rejoining the experience. On top of it all, it gave me some of my best friends in the world, which in and of itself would have made all the ridicule worth it.

Oh, and one last thing. Yes, it's extremely fake.

FAN FICTION
"Opening Up a Fandom: Choose Your Destiny"
by Julia Siciliano

I have been reading since I was two years old, driven by a burning need to know whatever insights could be gleaned from the pages of the books ... and magazines... and newspapers... that seemed so mesmerizing to adults everywhere. Of course, it would be a good many years before this reasoning would, or could, be articulated, and several additional years before this need could be refined into an interest not only in what was happening, but in why it occurred.

I envisioned critical junctures and key decisions, the outcomes of which could change the fate of the universe. How much of our world was coincidence and how much of our existence was a direct result of choices made by fallible humans? Hindsight, as they say, is 20/20- but what if decisions and outcomes could be mapped with a degree of certainty that could help us in selecting the right path? What insight could be gained by modeling the past against a decision-outcome matrix, rating and ranking our choices against what is best for self, others, state, country, and planet? Certainly such a device would be a game-changer in politics and warfare, not to mention further accelerating the pace of innovation and change. The individual who could monetize such a thing would be wealthy beyond their wildest dreams – or perhaps not, as such an outcome would surely have been predicted should the device work as intended.

Back in 80s, I knew nothing of the theories of infinite universes or multiverses that complimented my interests, I knew nothing of chaos theory, nor any of the physics behind those theories. What I did know was a series of books that would change my outlook and perspective on life, and the opportunities that present themselves: Edward Packard's *Choose Your Own Adventure* series. Marketed to younger readers, the books allowed the reader to make choices for the characters that then altered the narrative's actions and outcomes. Two readers of the same book could have two very different stories and endings depending on the choices made by the reader throughout the book, and as each novella was released I was determined to map all possible timelines and outcomes to ensure I could read the story with the most satisfying plot and conclusion possible. *If you choose to enter the cave, turn to page 76! If you decide to play it safe and return home, turn to page 200!*

As a voracious reader, I quickly read my way through the entire series and would wait, eager for each month's trip to the bookstore to see whether there was a new addition to the lineup. All too often, there was not, so I would content myself with books from other series, or standalone novels, or really – anything I could cajole my father into purchasing for me. Still, though, I was rarely satisfied with the choices the characters made, or how the plots concluded. It seemed to me that people could have been much better versions of themselves than they were written to be, and too often were their own worst enemy. Was it poor writing, or a reflection of reality? The answer, I am sure, was a bit of both – contrivances based on a caricature of the real world, placed to move the plot along to its inevitable conclusion – but I would find myself daydreaming of more palatable endings. If only Elizabeth had chosen to mention how uncomfortable she was instead of going along with her friends, tragedy could have been averted! If Collin had spoken out in favor of Mr. Jacobs' proposal, he would have been on the fast track for a scholarship instead of working odd jobs!

One day, I came to a realization, courtesy of Dolly Parton and her song 9 to 5. In trying to pinpoint for a friend why exactly I despised the song, I inadvertently highlighted where my predilection for *Choose Your Own Adventure* came from. I hated – HATED – the thought of someone letting things happen TO them, rather than making things happen. The passiveness of living in a manner where the world and external forces inflict indignities and remove opportunities was anathema to me. I wanted to be in charge of my own outcomes. I wanted to write my own destiny. I wanted to make things happen- and in doing so, I could control my path in life. If I didn't like it – I could change it.

Putting this into effect started off slowly, though. Before I was mature enough to live it personally, I had to live it vicariously through the stories I read and the heroes within. As a child, I was very much into the Nancy Drew mystery stories, having been gifted the entire set from my mother's childhood collection. I distinctly recall discussing one of Nancy's pre-dicaments with my mother, explaining why it didn't make sense and how the entire story would have been different if Nancy had only left a note for her housekeeper Hannah as she had intended to do. My mother semi-patiently explained that there wouldn't have been a story if people always did the logical thing. This bothered me, so I spent the next few hours writing up a better ending, one that I could relate to. While I was at it, I figured, I might as well remove some of the supporting characters' more annoying traits and tics that had manifested as expressions of stereotypes. The resultant re-write was amateur and childish, and I absolutely adored it. It felt right.

Fan Fiction

As I got older, and grew attached to and invested in various fandoms, I found myself with a dilemma. While I still wanted to see my favorite characters involved in meaningful plot lines with empowering outcomes, I lacked both the time to spend doing my own re-writes, and the desire to take away from myself the joy of discovering where a story was headed. Still, there had to be a way to accomplish what I was looking for.

Around this time, I counted myself as a fan of three main fan-verses: *Buffy the Vampire Slayer*, *X-Files*, and Harry Potter. I spent more time than I should admit poking around online forums and spoiler sites, theory and origin story discussion groups, and finally, buried deep in someone's signature line, I saw a link that grabbed my attention. It was a simple one liner, advertising that the final chapter of the 4th Harry Potter book was posted and available for download. My heart quickened: was I about to read an illicit pirated copy of a book that wasn't due to be released for another 6 months?

Of course, as I quickly determined, it wasn't a pirated version of Rowling's work. It was a fan-written Harry Potter book 4. Tired of waiting, literarily-inclined fans (and some not-so-inclined!) had taken to writing their own installments, from short stories to entire alternate novels. Down into the rabbit hole I went, finding entire websites that were searchable archives of fan-written stories (or fan-fic, as it has become known). Here were communities of people who felt as I did – that the stories our fandoms were serving up didn't quite meet our standards for one reason or another. Of course, not everyone shared my reasons for looking for different outcomes. Some people just wanted to have stories with different romantic pairings, or different characters (hence bringing forth the unfortunate trope of the

"Mary Sue", aka writing yourself into the action, often quite disjointedly and illogically). Others asked the same question I did: what would have happened IF... what paths opened up for the characters if different choices were made? What were the possibilities that manifested for the continuation of a story beyond what the original creator intended? By extending the fandom's universe with fan-written stories, the characters become more personalized, more three-dimensional, because readers were selecting story arcs that aligned with topics and paths that specifically resonated with him- or herself. Imaginations were stoked; conversations about archetypes, themes, motivations, and historical parallels developed. Friendships were formed. Fan followings sprang up for particularly talented fan-fiction authors who added meaningful, narrative-driven stories featuring beloved characters, allowing fans to spend just a little more time in a fictional world. And for some of us – well, we got the ability to choose our own adventure, and play in a fandom that was deeper and richer than ever imagined by the original creator. As for me, I try to live by my motto and "make things happen!" in my personal and professional life, but when I have a little bit of free time for some escapism, I still go back and seek out fiction that takes those characters I loved and allows one more spin behind the wheel, one more opportunity to explore what happens IF....

A door gets opened, and beyond is an expanded universe of infinite possibility. If you choose to walk through the door, turn to page 195. If you choose to walk away, go ahead and continue to the next page, but remember – there is a fandom out there for everyone, and if it can be dreamed, someone, somewhere has probably written a story about it. With heartfelt thanks to those fan fiction authors from back in the day who led me through many doors (and a window or two!): B.L. Purdom, the inimitable Bonetree, and Isabelle, among other notables — none of whom I have ever met or spoken to, but all of whom have inspired me in one way or another.

PERIOD DRAMAS
"Ringing the Period Drama Klaxon"
by Amanda-Rae Prescott

I must confess that the only bachelorette party I have ever attended was for a fictional character. While many Americans spent the Friday of Labor Day weekend in 2015 at barbeques or at the beach, I attended a stag night party for Mrs. Hughes from *Downton Abbey* at the Sheraton Hotel in Atlanta. That weekend over 50,000 nerds flooded the city to attend Dragon*Con, one of the biggest multi-genre conventions in America. I was dressed as the female version of Jack Ross, the black jazz singer who had a guest stint during season 4. Two women (plus a doll) in Mrs. Hughes' severe black dresses with chatelaines dangling from their waist were sipping from phallic shaped straws.

Unfortunately, I couldn't stay for the whole thing because I had to change into a Joan Harris costume for the *Mad Men* meetup at the top of the Westin Peachtree. On the 72nd floor, which rotates around so you can see the entire Atlanta skyline, Don and Megan Draper along with Roger Sterling and Jessica Rabbit were also in attendance. We had a few drinks and appetizers and the conversation drifted very quickly away from *Mad Men* so I headed back to the other event. When I came back to the Sheraton, the *Downton Abbey* cosplayers were between tipsy and drunk. They moved into the lobby next to the bar. Thomas Barrow and Jimmy were pretending to be Chippendales giving Lady Edith a lap dance.

Even though I am not much of a partier usually, it was an amazing feeling to spend an evening at a convention away from traditional geek culture, getting to meet people and hang out with friends who shared my

Period Dramas

goals of making period drama fandom a bigger phenomenon. Although both *Downton Abbey* and *Mad Men* attracted considerable mainstream attention, both fandoms lacked elements of more traditional geek fandoms. While I was, yet again, the only nerd of color there, I was an equal in fandom. No one was judging my obsessions, likes or dislikes.

The road towards the fake bachelorette party and accepting that I needed to find the people who shared my interests was a long one. I was born into a family of Caribbean immigrants to America. Appreciation of British pop culture was inculcated in me from an early age. My family refused to install cable for religious reasons in the 90s. New York's PBS station Thirteen filled in massive gaps in my education and my entertainment. I also adored watching the documentaries on everything from ancient Egypt to the history of the Civil Rights movement. Curling up on the couch to watch *Masterpiece Theater* (now called *Masterpiece*) with my Mom was the best part of the week. Moving from one era to another each Sunday night was quite exciting.

Although I was doomed to a life of social isolation, I secretly enjoyed going against the grain with my choices. It didn't matter that no one in school shared my obsession with the 18th century and other eras of history. My teachers rewarded my intense interest with high grades on tests and essays. The knowledge I gained from watching a PBS program could often be applied to the topic at hand. The past, from the ancient world through the 1970s, shaped my imagination. While many people were inspired by superheroes and fairy tales, I found my inspiration in those characters I met on *Masterpiece Theatre*. I pictured myself wearing pretty costumes across the centuries, striking up conversations with Mr. Darcy, or plotting royal intrigues. When I was in a more serious mood, I pictured what my life would have actually been like in the days of slavery or colonialism. It would be many years before I would learn to sew for myself, but I made a careful study of the costumes in all of those productions.

I wish someone had told me back then that all of my attitudes were signs of geeky behavior and of being on the autism spectrum. I didn't like Batman or Captain America, not in the comics or in the cartoons. I only played the video games that came preloaded on the old school Macs. All of the 1990s anime, manga, and other Japanese pop culture trends made no sense to me. I wasn't into science fiction, fantasy, or horror either. I skipped all of the most popular TV shows from those genres. Mom was disappointed I couldn't get into *Star Wars*. My love of period dramas would remain, for many years, a solo pursuit.

The first definitive step towards realizing my period drama nerd potential occurred while watching the 2002 remake of *The Forsyte Saga*. This was the first period drama which forms a clear picture in my head. I was old enough to fully appreciate the entire scope of the story. I remember being glued to the old wooden panel TV, feeling sorry for Irene. I made it a point to make sure I caught every part of the miniseries. My Mom was just as hooked, although Grandma was convinced that the 1969 version was better. Arguing over which adaptation is better is an important part of the period drama fandom experience.

In my freshman year of high school I joined my first fandom. Although *House M.D.* was a modern drama, it was incredibly helpful in a few ways for expanding my interests. I discovered groups and blogs for period drama fans and Anglophiles. These online groups and blogs gave me hope that one day

Period Dramas

I would find friends in real life to share my interests with. The main fandoms in my large public high school in the mid-2000s were bands, *The Lord of the Rings* and anime. People at school no longer made fun of my interests, but many were unaware of my favorite period dramas. My after school and weekend chats with fans across America and the world helped me get through the stress of homework. In between *House M.D.* seasons, there were online group watching sessions devoted to Hugh Laurie's previous works. These events led me to discover the period comedies *Jeeves and Wooster* and *BlackAdder*. After years of crying over depressing scenes, here were two side-splitting funny period pieces. Laurie's crazy antics as Bertie Wooster led me to binge reading P.G. Wodehouse's short stories based on 1920s and 1930s Britain. As a child I adored the historical satire cartoon *Hysteria*, and I was delighted to see an adult version of the concept on *BlackAdder.* Both are on my all-time favorites list.

Discovering *Doctor Who* in the fall of 2007 was the final piece in the puzzle of finding friends in real life that shared my period drama interests. I told my classmate in my freshman African Literature class that I was really obsessed with *House M.D.* She suggested trying out *Doctor Who* because it had a lot for Anglophiles to love. Seeing Christopher Eccleston fight off aliens in the episode "Rose" changed my life in several ways. I finally found the thing that made me a traditional nerd. More importantly, it was my entry into the world of meetups at comic cons and official premieres. These events were excellent networking possibilities. Conversations that started as compliments on my Martha Jones or Amy Pond cosplays led to admissions that people loved the 1970s series *Upstairs, Downstairs* and other classics.

Downton Abbey first aired on PBS on December 18, 2011. I knew from the moment the pilot aired that this show was the start of the next big thing in period dramas. I was instantly enthralled with watching the lives of the Crawley family and their household staff. The characters were a microcosm of bigger developments in the Edwardian and World War I era. *Downton Abbey* was the first time I joined a period drama fandom as the episodes were airing. On a whim I entered the contest for fans to attend a preview screening of the second season with the cast in Manhattan in December 2012. I didn't have much hope but I wanted to try anyway. While I was at a holiday party for my job at the time, I got an email saying I won the contest. I screamed out loud in the middle of the party. I felt like I struck Powerball! I was an awkward mess because I drank more of the free champagne than I was used to but I still had a fabulous time. That night was my first ever meetup for a period drama fandom. I finally found the thrilling feeing I get from meeting fellow cosplayers or fans at a comic con in a different genre entirely. Once my closest friends from *Doctor Who* fandom discovered *Downton Abbey*, the good feelings continued to grow. I live tweeted episode reactions every Sunday night. I reviewed episodes on multiple blogs. I managed to attend the premieres for seasons 4, 5, and 6. These happy experiences cemented my pride in being a period drama geek.

The benefits of narrowing my focus and fully immersing myself in the world of period dramas were many. The years of social isolation for my interests was finally over. I solidified my outlet for my love of history and overactive imagination. I had friends in real life and online to complain to about plot twists with. I also expanded my experiences from *Doctor Who* cosplay into new areas of costuming.

Period Dramas

For years I put off taking sewing lessons out of sheer laziness. eBay had all the U.K. designer brands I needed to assemble a Clara Oswald cosplay. Vintage shops had *Mad Men* and *Downton Abbey* inspired pieces. My inspiration to reverse that trend came from an unexpected place. Watching the first few episodes of the new *Poldark* series in late June 2015 gave me the burst of inspiration I finally needed to learn how to sew. I fell madly in love with Demelza Poldark's simple country wedding dress. I pictured myself walking around a comic convention wearing a late 18th Century brick red cotton round gown. I made a call to the vintage sewing machine repair shop to fix my Grandma's machines and a trip to Joann Fabrics to translate the vision in my head into supplies. As I cut out the pieces in the pattern, I didn't realize how much I already knew about clothing construction from years of cosplay. When I came to an unfamiliar term on the pattern, I turned to YouTube. Nine days later, I finished the dress. I finally turned my childhood dreams of wearing the dresses I saw on screen into reality. A working class dress was a far cry from my childhood imagination of wearing royal robes but that touch of irony was the motivation I needed to learn as much as I could about historical costuming.

My journey in *Poldark* fandom started as merely a desire for distraction. I didn't intend for the show to influence my cosplay or become the first fandom where I was able to take an active role in building a community. In the spring of 2015, I was busy working on my journalism Master's thesis and I was yearning for stress relief between research and interview stints. I first heard of *Poldark* in 2008. There was a special that counted down the 12 best *Masterpiece Theatre* programs from the beginning in the early 1970s until that point. I lost track of the series until spring of 2015, when I found out that

161

Aidan Turner from *Being Human* was leading the remake of *Poldark* which was airing on PBS in June. I decided to give myself the rare opportunity to start a period drama by reading the source material and the older adaptation first. In all 3 versions, Ross Poldark's life as a miner in late 18th Century Cornwall allowed me to view my favorite century in history from a new vantage point. Very few dramas focus on Britain after the loss of the Revolutionary War and the following depression and conflicts with France. In between the politics, the unlikely romance of Ross and Demelza, plus family drama, added to my enjoyment of all versions of the story.

Cultivating a deeper love of historical costuming increased my enjoyment of period drama fandom fourfold. I finally had a roadmap for learning how to sew period correct attire. Learning the differences between screen accurate or replicating the costumes seen on TV or movies and the construction methods of the period was an important step.

Poldark fandom was the first time I played a role in shaping the community of a period drama fandom. I turned my love of the costumes into the Poldark Costuming Project, a Tumblr blog devoted to analyzing the costumes featured on each episode. Slowly but surely, more people are expressing interest in making both historically accurate attire based on the era and cosplay from the show.

After cutting my teeth on the simple dresses of *Poldark*, I turned my attention to more daunting 18th Century designs. I first encountered *Outlander* after a few friends dragged me to the New York Comic Con panel for the graphic novel *The Exile* in 2010. After realizing that it was more of a historical novel and romance than science fiction/fantasy, I made sure to read every book available at the time. The advent of the series on Starz

Period Dramas

turned into a boon for cosplay inspiration. Season premieres and convention panels became my personal runway as I was eager to tackle the more complicated French and Scottish 18th Century styles. After *Outlander*, I turned my attentions towards replicating Angelica Schuyler from the musical *Hamilton*. Translating theater costumes into cosplay was a breeze. Cosplaying Angelica was also a handy excuse to burst out into song in the hallway at New York Comic Con.

Along with networking and costuming opportunities, getting more involved allowed to me to mitigate the number one frustration of being a period drama geek. It is pretty inevitable you will look to the U.K, Europe, Canada, and Australia as the main sources for television period dramas. For every *John Adams*, there are way more modern or genre dramas. Unlike *Sherlock* on *Masterpiece*, the period dramas do not have same day as U.K. airing contracts. The wait for US networks or streaming sites such as Netflix and Amazon Prime to air period dramas ranges from 3 weeks to years depending on the contract. Connecting with fellow fans on Facebook groups, Twitter, and Tumblr helps US fans get the episodes at the same time as the UK fans. Waiting for the US airing often means missing opportunities for active participation in fandom or seeing spoilers online. In order to mitigate the potential ethical and legal issues, most period drama fans watch the UK versions online and then the American airing.

Coupled with significant airing delays is often the absence of promotional events and US press coverage. A few weeks ago, I signed a petition which eventually gained over 500 signatures asking PBS to improve their *Poldark* PR efforts in the States. *Downton Abbey* had very good representation in the US, but many of the newer U.K. period dramas haven't had anywhere near a quarter of the attention.

This isn't to say that Hollywood is completely incapable of producing period dramas. I discovered *Mad Men* a few months before *Downton Abbey* and chances are very high it will still show up in "Best TV Shows Of All Time" lists 10 years from now. Although many consider *Outlander* a U.K. period drama, the writers are American. Movies that are movie/play/musical adaptations and biopics tend to dominate US period dramas. On US television, current trends are towards inserting supernatural elements in period pieces or covering the 1970s-1990s which, to me, is too close to current. Another trend is towards quick cancellations. Within the last few months, *Mercy Street* on PBS and *Underground* on WGN America were cancelled from broadcast TV. Although both dealt with slavery and freedom around the Civil War era, *Mercy Street* lost too much money for the investors and *Underground* suffered from a regime change at the network. Similarly, Amazon recently pulled the plug on *Z: The Beginning of Everything*, *The Good Girls Revolt,* and *The Last Tycoon*. The current reasoning is that all 3 cost too much money for too little return. These trends influence period drama geeks to look elsewhere, especially if they prefer television to film.

Although I was very comfortable in sharing "Evil Butler Barrow" memes on Twitter, there are times that I began to doubt my self-imposed fandom isolation. Quite a few of my *Doctor Who* and *Sherlock* friends didn't share my intense desire and narrow focus. They were persistent in attempts to persuade me to watch their favorites, but they failed. The questions swirled around my head. Why weren't more people watching period dramas without supernatural or mythological elements? Why won't the media give my favorite period dramas more PR attention? How dare my friends from *Downton Abbey* fandom dabble in fandoms outside of period dramas?

I still didn't care about superheroes, even as they became increasingly popular. I was too horrified by the violence in the pilot episode of *Game of Thrones* to watch more than 10 minutes. Anime and video games continue to elude my understanding. I knew what I liked and what I wanted to see from my fandom: more interactions between people. Period drama fans tend to enjoy their favorite shows in isolation. Encouraging online discussion and meetups became my long-term goal. There would be opportunities and obstacles that would prevent networking but the effort was well worth it.

There is one notable exception to my overall disdain for most mainstream fandom trends. *Hamilton* is the pop culture phenomenon that keeps on giving. I first read the biography *Alexander Hamilton* by Ron Chernow when it was first published in 2004. While most people didn't know yet, the life of the bastard orphan who built America's financial system was incredibly compelling. For many years I expected a miniseries to use Chernow's research for inspiration. Hearing the soundtrack for the first time made me feel an intense joy that Hamilton's life story was finally being told. My reading and citing of Hamilton's "Farmer Refuted" articles in my undergraduate senior project finally paid off. So many more people are passionate about early American history because of the cast recording and seeing *Hamilton* live. I wasn't fortunate enough to see the original cast of *Hamilton* but I managed to get into "The Room Where It Happened" on the same night the PBS documentary *Hamilton's America* aired on PBS. Seeing Javier Munoz belt out "My Shot" was as close to a religious experience as I will ever get on Broadway.

The frustrations from outside forces were easily overcome but the internal fandom battles are a lot more trying. Most of the period drama fandoms online have internal battles over "shipping" or arguments over the plot. Some have divisions between fans of the original source material (or older TV/movie editions) and fans of the newer adaptation. Some fandoms also have battles between people who favor a strict historical interpretation and those who prefer adding modernization or creative license. I ran into trouble on these fronts in both *Outlander* and *Poldark* fandoms and realized that the easiest solution is to either stay out of contentious debates or to find the people who agree with you and talk amongst yourselves.

The truly dark side of period drama fandom comes out when there are discussions on increasing diversity in Hollywood or the UK acting industry. I have engaged in many unsuccessful attempts to educate white period drama fans when this issue comes up in the period drama groups. Many fans of period dramas have bought into false historical narratives or haven't challenged their intrinsic belief in whiteness as the default, or even in some cases white supremacy. They don't realize how much of the history of racial minorities has been covered over or ignored. I have seen quite a few people openly state that "black people didn't exist back then". There have also been many people who make excuses about how productions would lose money if they pander to certain audiences or sanitize history. Some even try to justify all white casting by claiming the author of a fictional novel wanted historical accuracy. These arguments are nothing more than attempts to justify the status quo. For some reason it is harder for period drama fans to believe that Sophie Okonedo playing Margaret of Anjou in *The Hollow Crown*

Period Dramas

is ok than for them to believe the Anjou family myth that they are descendants of swans.

I have not had the same kind of racist pushback when it comes to cosplaying white characters from period dramas. The cast and crew I have met so far from my favorite while in costume have appreciated my work. So far, I have photos with Phyllis Logan from *Downton Abbey*, Caitriona Baife plus Terry Dresbach from *Outlander* and Robin Ellis from the 1970s *Poldark*. People may confuse me for "Merida's cousin" but I have never had an incident where I was mocked for my skin color. I am not sure if it's because the trolls haven't found me yet or that the fans I encounter truly believe that cosplay is for everyone.

Ignoring diverse audiences these days spells doom for the entire genre over time. Potential viewers are alienated and stories are ignored by default. In theory, anyone can watch any TV show or movie they want. Anyone can form an emotional connection to a character. In reality, the lack of diverse storytelling is a turnoff for audiences of color. No matter how pretty the 1810s countryside in *Emma* is, people will not have characters that look like them to relate to. Casting with an eye to racial diversity is only part of the overall solution. Many people want to see new period dramas tackle regions and topics beyond the 20th Century or slavery in America. Issues such as racism, colonialism, and ethnic identity can be explored without American-centric bias. More minority directors, writers, cinematographers, and producers would also go a long way towards moving things forward. Period drama fans who perpetuate regressive attitudes about the genre alienate potential viewers. The same concept applies to issues of representation of gender, sexuality, and other areas of diversity as well.

These arguments strangely enough do not extend to period theater productions. Most people are comfortable with theater productions casting whomever is available to act. *Hamilton* fandom is important to me for more than the history. The insistence on casting actors of color for white historical figures fulfilled a dream of mine. For many years, I wanted a miniseries that would feature diverse actors in the 18th Century that didn't involve slavery. While the 2013 U.K. movie *Belle* had a biracial woman as the lead character, the US promotion was lackluster. Finally, there was a show on Broadway with people who looked like me. And yet the show also brilliantly referenced the struggle for freedom from slavery. Cosplaying Angelica Schuyler has been a wonderful opportunity because I don't need to alter much about my natural appearance to look like the character. Little kids at conventions recognize me instantly. One day they might be period drama nerds too.

Despite all of the online arguments and the side eyes from other nerds, I have had a bounty of good experiences. Diving deep into my interests has paid off for me intellectually and emotionally. If you're someone who has been binging *Lark Rise to Candleford* and wondering where the other period drama geeks are, we're just one search away on Google or Facebook!

STAR TREK
"Highly Logical, Boldly Emotional"
by Erik Henriksen

I am not a Trekkie.

I have been desperately asserting this for years using a simple checklist. I do not go to conventions. I do not wear Vulcan ears or have a Starfleet uniform tucked away in my closet. I do not own autographed photos of any *Star Trek* actors. I do not pontificate on the disadvantages of bioneural gel packs versus standard isolinear circuitry. Naturally, this exhaustive "not-a-trekkie" checklist confirms that I'm not the stereotypical *Star Trek* fan but rather a normal guy who just happens to like *Star Trek*. Who happens to like *Star Trek* a lot. Of course, when I'm not engaged in self-deluding mental checklists, I recognize this is absolute nonsense.

The truth is I have been snobbishly setting myself above Trekkies for so long, I reflexively ignore the indicative signs of Trekkieness. I do not go to conventions but I have been part of a virtual Starfleet crew. I do not wear Vulcan ears but I have worn a Romulan forehead prosthesis. I do not have a Starfleet uniform but I do own an adult-size Starfleet pajama onesie. I do not own any autographed photos of *Star Trek* actors but if I did, they would be framed and displayed proudly on the walls of my man-cave. I do not pontificate on the disadvantages of bioneural gel packs over isolinear chips but I do have a well-researched opinion on the matter that I would be happy to share if anyone thought to ask me. As an added evidential bonus, I admit that I might also own a toy Romulan Warbird with light up nacelles and four button array of activated action sounds. Romulan disruptor fire is like music to my ears.

169

Erik Henriksen

The obvious hypocrisy notwithstanding, I do genuinely believe that my love of *Star Trek* goes beyond simple "fanboy". Whether I fit the "Trekkie" label, I like to think that my infatuation with *Star Trek* is somewhat sophisticated. I believe that if one watches *Star Trek* with an erudite eye, each episode offers something for your heart, your head and your soul that not only entertains but also elevates.

My earliest vivid memory of *Star Trek* involves the opening scene of *Star Trek: the Motion Picture* wherein the Klingons mount a futile attack against a mysterious energy cloud that had invaded their space. I was thirteen years old when I first experienced this scene. I had previously watched episodes from the Original Series, of course – but my first *emotional* connection with *Star Trek* was brought on by those three Klingon battlecruisers bearing down on the massive blue energy cloud. In describing the beauty and brilliance of this opening scene, there is a lot to unpack. First, the camera angles used in the initial moments of the scene to follow the course of these ships on approach to unknown enemy was like nothing I had seen before. The intense portrayal of Mark Lenard's Klingon commander is in perfect sync with the enthralling musical score by Jerry Goldsmith. I once read a review of the scene by Jeff Bond (Geek Monthly) in which he brilliantly observed that the Klingon commander's barked orders and quick, downward hand thrusts are so well timed with the score that it is almost as if the Klingon commander is conducting the music in some way. Just think about that for a moment. To achieve that kind of synergy, either the acting had to be choreographed with the music or the music had to be written note-by-note for the acting. Beyond the excellent cinematography, the brilliant acting and beautiful score that drew me into the scene, the very futility of the Klingons' efforts to defeat this mysterious enemy also left a lasting impression on my thirteen-year old mind. Halfway through the scene, it becomes obvious that the Klingons are no match for the invading energy cloud. If they do not withdraw, they will be vaporized by the crackling energy weapons launched at them by the cloud. Nevertheless, they persist; only years later when the Klingons make several more appearances on the *Next Generation* did I understand why they could not give up the fight. After the seven-minute scene concluded, I was feeling admiration for the Klingons' bravery, sorrow for the tragedy that had just played out, curiosity about the identity of whatever was at the center of that mysterious cloud and concern for those still in its path. The overlapping and intersecting thoughts and emotions brought out in me by this scene seemed just as well choreographed as the scene itself. From that moment on, I was in love with *Star Trek* as each of the movies and episodes that followed in later years brought me back again and again to that initial experience at age 13.

I have often reflected on what it is about *Star Trek* that resonates with me. When telling any story, success is measured by how effectively it connects and influences the audience. I am not a marketing guy but I understand there is a long-standing debate about whether appeals to our emotions or appeals to our intellect are more effective when influencing people. Brands have historically targeted our emotions to get the biggest bang for their marketing buck because they know that emotions drive behavior. Look no further than our annual Super Bowl commercials which typically leave you laughing or crying or both. I remember one particularly absurd commercial that left me almost in tears that I couldn't explain. In GM's "Robot" commercial from 2007, a robotic arm on the assembly line messes up, gets fired, leaves the company, wanders the streets, fails at several subsequent odd jobs and eventually attempts suicide only to wake up and realize it was only a nightmare. It bears mentioning that this little melodrama plays out to the ballad "All By Myself" by Eric Carmen. I found myself genuinely sad for the robot, amused at the absurdity and mad that I was feeling anything at all because "how stupid was that, anyway?" Strong emotions leave lasting impressions.

Of course, when making sound decisions our society supports the rational approach over the emotional. Rational thinking has deep roots in western society going all the way back to the Greeks. Accused criminals are innocent until proven guilty. Scientific facts begin as scientific theories. Intellectual arguments are applauded while outbursts of emotion are often dismissed as "not helpful." While currently under attack by fringe elements, intellect and rationality remain central to what we value – impartial justice, scholarly pursuits, facts that trump feelings and allow for sound decision-making. For my part, I fall perfectly in line with these values. I gravitate toward intellectuals and like to spend time thinking about things. I'm committed to learning and make it a part of my daily life. Case in point, I'm addicted to documentaries in the same way others are addicted to sports. In one particularly memorable episode of the TV show *Frasier*, Martin sits down with Frasier to watch a documentary called *Lost on a Mountain*. Martin begins to aggravate Frasier with a cacophony of sounds as he settles into his squeaky chair and tears into a bag of pretzels. Frasier erupts with rage, whereupon Martin suggests he go watch his documentary somewhere else. Frasier quips: "Just what do you suggest – that I find a documentary bar and watch it on their big screen?" The suggestion is absurd, of course, and that's why it's funny. But I would go to that bar. I would seriously go to that bar. Stories that stir our imaginations and allow us to expand our minds can be very compelling.

Finally, healthy humans have an ethical center. We acknowledge the difference between right and wrong and are hopefully guided by a solid set of shared principles. When presented with an ethical dilemma, many of us strive to do the right thing. Finding our moral center is something that a good upbringing can reinforce, but to me our ethics seem more instinctual than acquired. My own morality constantly yearns for confirmation. Some seek that confirmation from religious institutions while others follow a philosophical path to enlightenment but no matter how we come by our spiritual pearls of wisdom, we do our best to critically examine our own choices while attempting to avoid passing judgment on the choices of others. To navigate this moral complexity, we often seek assistance from a variety of sources like self-help books, conversations with our friends and family, religious texts, the preacher's sermon or even movies and television. The soul needs its soup.

Circling back to *Star Trek*, like any proper fan I have watched each of the *Star Trek* movies several dozen times. I've seen every episode of the Original Series, *The Next Generation*, *Deep Space Nine*, *Voyager* and *Enterprise*. I've seen my favorite episodes several dozen times. I found something different to love in each series. While not my favorite, I cherish TOS (the Original Series) for the way it challenged the social norms of the day with its progressive values. I loved *The Next Generation* for its emphasis on peace and diplomacy. *Deep Space Nine* touched on matters of faith and conflict in an epic fashion that I found thrilling. *Voyager* explored what would happen when highly-developed principles are challenged by the need to survive in a way that reminded me of *Lord of the Flies*. Finally, *Enterprise* showed us how independent cultures could overcome long-standing rivalries and come together in common cause.

These predominant themes make for great entertainment but they hardly serve to put *Star Trek* on a pedestal above the cornucopia of science fiction that has hit the airwaves over the last fifty years. *Star Trek* has had stiff competition with similar formats for decades: *Space 1999, Lost in Space, Doctor Who, Buck Rogers, Battlestar Galactica, Babylon 5, Firefly, Farscape,* and the many iterations of *Stargate* to name just a few. Do not get me started on the *Star Trek* versus *Star Wars* debate. Okay, fine. There is no point in comparing *Star Trek* to *Star Wars* as they occupy two distinct, adjacent and mutually inclusive spots in my heart. Suffice to say, gaining immortal and iconic status in our culture requires something special but rising above the competition requires something unique – a differentiator that resonates with us more than any of the other shows that compete for our love.

For me, *Star Trek* has mastered a multidimensional technique that appeals to my heart, stimulates my mind and speaks to my soul in equal measure, often in the same episode. To put it another way, a single episode can feature a thought-provoking scientific breakdown of a spatial anomaly, a heartbreaking personal loss by one of the characters, a flashy and epic battle between starships and a surprisingly relevant ethical dilemma. The juxtaposition of these elements is often flawlessly woven together in just over 40 minutes – not always, but often.

An example of this from the Original Series in an episode called "A Taste of Armageddon." The *Enterprise* makes contact with a world that is at war with a neighboring world. The leader of this world informs Kirk and crew that the two planets have learned to avoid the complete devastation of war because computers are used. When a "hit" is scored by one of the planets, the people declared "dead" willingly walk into antimatter chambers and are vaporized. Anan 7 further tells Kirk that his ship and all the crew aboard her have been declared casualties and will be executed. When Kirk flatly refuses, the landing party members are taken prisoner. Naturally, our heroes escape and destroy the war simulation computers. Kirk proudly declares that before the planets can find peace, they must truly experience the horrors of war. Clearly the message was anti-war but the scenario was so absurd that it forced me to decide which method was better: quiet, painless execution or violent, agonizing death in battle? The painless death would seem preferable but it was so cold and calculated with no heart and no glory. To this day, I still cannot decide if Kirk did the right thing.

The Next Generation also offered a bounty of great episodes. Some episodes are beautiful and haunting like "Inner Light" wherein Captain Picard is probed by an alien device that causes him to live out an entire lifetime on another planet while he lay unconscious on the *Enterprise* bridge. He falls in love, has children and grandchildren, and lives his whole life all in the span of a few minutes in real time. When he wakes up, he learns that everyone he knew and loved on this far away planet are mere memories stored by this ancient probe whose purpose is to preserve the memories of a dying planet. Can you imagine waking up from *your life* to discover that it was all someone else's memories? Everyone you have loved for the past few decades have been dead for a thousand years? Even though I was fully prepared for Picard's snap back to reality, I remember feeling stunned at the end of it.

Erik Henriksen

One of my favorite TNG episodes is "The Best of Both Worlds" in which the crew of the Enterprise confronts and defeats an invading Borg cube in epic fashion. This two-part episode is packed with powerful story elements. First, few antagonists evoke fear and horror quite like the Borg and their infamous introduction: "We are the Borg. Lower your shields and surrender your ships. We will add your biological and technological distinctiveness to our own. Your culture will adapt to service us. Resistance is futile." A chilling message to be sure but we witness first-hand just how serious and even predictive this declaration can be. The Borg are not bluffing. They have destroyed hundreds of cultures, many in a single day. They are relentless and unstoppable. Ironically, the terrifying confrontation in this episode is used almost as a backdrop for the real story. When Captain Picard gets abducted and assimilated by the Borg, his first officer Commander Riker must step up and fend off the Borg invasion. Can Riker make the hard decisions or would he buckle under the pressure? Story aside, the episode is set to an ominous musical score and thrilling special effects. In the final scene of part one, Captain Picard steps out of the shadows to reveal his assimilation. His grey skin is covered in motorized devices and there is a mechanical tone to his words. As the music crescendos, he looks directly into the camera whereupon the laser mounted to the side of his head seems to pierce through the television and into our eyes. Just as your heart is pounding in your chest, preparing your body for the inevitable battle, the scene goes dark followed by the dreaded "To be continued..." I can only imagine the screams ringing out in thousands of households across the country when the episode aired live.

Star Trek

I must admit that the testosterone-driven man-child inside me lives for epic space battles. I tend to grin from ear to ear when I see two ships engaged in battle, photon torpedoes smashing against energy shields, the bridge crew being thrown across our field of vision in a haze of sparks and smoke. If you make that a fleet of ships flying in formation against another fleet of ships, the resulting carnage will have me foaming at the mouth. I confess that it is carnal and primitive. I'm not proud of it. Despite a slow start, *Deep Space Nine* rewarded my early patience with some truly satisfying space battles. I remember sitting on my couch with a gaggle of friends when we first watched "The Way of the Warrior." Dozens of Klingon ships decloak and threaten a seemingly defenseless space station. After some obligatory posturing by the Klingons, Captain Sisko declares "I've got five thousand photon torpedoes armed and ready to launch." I noticed that the friend sitting on the couch to my left was crouched, on the balls of his feet as if he were getting ready to jump up and fire a phaser. Another friend was pacing behind us, chewing on his nails. The air in our tiny apartment living room was crackling with a nervous energy that promptly exploded when Sisko yelled "Fire!" Just as he promised, thousands of torpedoes started firing in every direction. The camera followed a few of the torpedoes to their targets which blew apart in satisfying fireballs. Our neighbors probably wondered if they were missing a football game because of the rowdy cheers that erupted from us. It certainly felt that exciting.

There were many other DS9 episodes with battles like that. But in between these nerdgasms, the series presented us with many fascinating intellectual challenges and moral dilemmas. It dives into the spiritual realm as the featured race is deeply religious but scarred by decades of brutal occupation. The series follows the political machinations of Kai Wynn who attains the highest religious position in Bajoran society. She uses religion to fulfill her political ambitions and there are many who get hurt in the process. It also grapples with the very hot topic of terrorism. To oust the brutal Cardassian occupation, everyday Bajorans become terrorists against the unwelcome regime. Are these acts of terrorism justified? Our societal upbringing tells us that terrorists are evil. The series forces me to reconcile this notion with the fact that the Bajoran protagonists were once terrorists themselves. Reexamining my moral stance on terrorism was delightfully unexpected and ultimately healthy.

It is hard to label any of the *Star Trek* series my favorite. Under duress, I must admit a special fondness for *Voyager*. I do love the innovation of a female captain. I also delight at the host of new aliens introduced from the Delta Quadrant. However, what draws me to this series more than any of the others are the twin concepts of home and family.

This series takes a lone Starfleet vessel and tosses it across the galaxy, 70,000 light years from home. Captain Janeway and the Voyager crew have been transported to the Delta Quadrant by an entity called "the Caretaker." It will take Voyager 75 years at maximum speed to get back home. At the end of the first episode, Captain Janeway does have the opportunity to use the Caretaker's technology to get her crew home but doing so will result in this powerful technology falling into the hands of the Kazon (some pretty bad dudes). Rather than allow an entire region of space to be threatened by the Kazon, Janeway destroys the technology and strands herself and the crew of Voyager in the Delta Quadrant.

Almost immediately, the crew of *Voyager* must make some difficult decisions. Survival in the Delta Quadrant might be made easier if the crew abandoned a few of the lofty principles upon which the Federation is founded upon. Trading useful technology to the locals would certainly gain them valuable resources but this would be a violation of the most basic tenets of Starfleet. Captain Janeway continuously acts as the conscience of Voyager by insisting that the crew remember who they are and where they come from. There were many episodes wherein the crew faced this decision. I couldn't help but be reminded of the Lord of the Flies with Captain Janeway as the optimistic and principled Ralph who never gave up on getting rescued but was never willing to sacrifice his humanity before that day arrived.

Every episode of *Voyager* centers around this pervasive and overwhelming desire to get back to the Alpha Quadrant and reunite with family. Voyager's mission to get home permeates every decision made throughout the seven seasons and yet over the course of those seven seasons, the crew of Voyager begins to realize that Voyager itself has become "home" and their fellow crewmates have become "family." When Voyager finally does get home in the final episode, I admit that at first, I felt it was too abrupt. I thought perhaps it was unplanned like so many other endings to great science fiction shows. One minute they're still stuck in the Delta Quadrant and the next minute, they are home and they live happily ever after. What the heck?

Upon reflection, I believe the final episode was anti-climactic because the mission to reach home and family had already been accomplished long before Voyager returned to the Alpha Quadrant. The deep connection that each member of the crew felt both to the ship and to each other had supplanted any connections they might have had before they were abducted by the Caretaker. *Star Trek Voyager* is special to me because it tapped into a personal truth of mine: "Home is where the heart is."

Finally, *Star Trek Enterprise* revived the franchise again by setting us back to a time before the Original Series, before the foundation of the Federation. Earthlings were just making their way into the galaxy with the help of their new friends, the Vulcans. At the beginning of this series, we feel alone and isolated...but hopeful. There is so much out there waiting for us to discover. The early episodes of *Enterprise* make you feel young and ready for anything. As the series progresses, each encounter gets Earth more and more entangled in galactic events. The Earthers just can't seem to stay out of everyone's business. At the same time, Captain Archer (played by the talented Scott Bakula) manages to make a lot of new friends and put Earth at the center of things. Just as we start to feel less alone and isolated, Earth is viciously attacked using a superweapon created by aliens called the Xindi. The next few seasons focus on a lonely mission into dangerous, unfamiliar space to avenge those killed in the first attack and prevent an Earth-ending second attack. The end of the series sees Captain Archer and the crew of Enterprise bringing together four alien races previously at each other's throats to create the United Federation of Planets. *Star Trek Enterprise* is a hopeful and optimistic series that imagines we are better together than we are apart – a notion that would seem to be more relevant than ever in these divisive times.

My love of *Star Trek* runs deep. It is firmly embedded in the experiences of my youth and its relevance in my life has been renewed again and again with each new series. The slow but steady character development causes me to become invested in the lives of these fictional characters. I admire Spock for his ability to balance his Vulcan discipline with his human heart. I want Commander Riker to be rewarded with his own ship someday but can't bear to see him missing from the bridge. I wonder how Garak is doing on the decimated world of Cardassia. I wish we could get updates on Tom and B'Elanna's baby girl. And I hope Doctor Phlox reconciles with his son someday. I am emotionally tied to these people that don't exist and I'm okay with that. The characters of *Star Trek* have captured my heart.

I'm fascinated by the science of *Star Trek* – not because the technology is impossible but rather because it is. In fact, the science of *Star Trek* which at the time seemed so fictional is proving to be predictive. Transparent aluminum from *Star Trek*: *the Voyage Home* now exists. It's called aluminum oxynitride. Most people now own a Starfleet hand-held communicator; we just call them cell phones. Medical hyposprays seemed awesome and impossible at the time but jet injection technology is here and in use. Tractor beams absolutely do not exist, right? Well, sort of. Optical tweezers use tiny lasers that can manipulate molecules. The list goes on. *Star Trek* is so predictive because the storytelling incorporates real science facts. Children inspired by the gadgets in *Star Trek* grow up to become scientists and engineers – and they try to build what inspires them. For me, *Star Trek* has spawned countless hours of thought and conjecture.

More than anything else, *Star Trek* challenges my moral assumptions. Most episodes tackle situations that range from familiar to absurd but wherever they fall on that continuum, these stories create a sort of petri dish wherein I can examine my assumptions about what is right and what is wrong. Our social constructs (religion, government and even family) all teach us there is a difference between right and wrong but the truth is the line between right and wrong is often blurred. Rather than declare right from wrong, *Star Trek* poses questions that inspire me to answer the questions myself after a lot of soul searching.

Star Trek has made me a better person for having watched it. It helps me empathize with others, it has opened my eyes to imagine a better future and inspires me to make thoughtful choices. I can only hope that future iterations of the franchise in the hands of the younger generations continue to tell stories that shape the lives of people like me. And I hope to still be around when *Star Trek* can be watched in a real life holosuite.

Live long and prosper, y'all.

MUSICAL THEATRE
"To Being an Us for Once, Instead of a Them"
by Stephen Webb

There are 525,600 minutes in a year. That means before my story really begins we have approximately 6,832,800 minutes of context that I have to provide. Don't worry. I'll give you the abridged version of that part.

I grew up in Douglasville, Georgia. It was pretty much exactly how you're thinking it was. As far back as I can remember, I was aware that the locals and I didn't see eye to eye on very much. I was the little 8 year old kid who was pulling for Michael Dukakis to win the 1988 Presidential election, despite everyone around me being conservatives. While my parents were listening to Conway Twitty, I was rhyming with the Beastie Boys. At holiday meals, while other people were talking about how much they loved hunting, I was sitting in a corner making snarky asides to my cousin about how it would be far more sporting if you offered the deer a rifle too. I never really felt like I fit in.

While fandom wasn't a thing that was actively encouraged specifically, the "geek" seeds were there. I played with my He-Man figures (I have still to this day never flown without that He-Man in my bag, but that is an entirely different essay). I remember being 5 years old and desperately trying to hit 88 mph on my big wheel, walking around my neighborhood with a plastic P.K.E. meter searching for ghosts, and as I got a bit older I even contemplated putting a bra on my head to create my very own Kelly LeBrock. Yet, I never had that one connection as a kid that defined or shaped who I was. I didn't see *Star Wars* until the 1997 re-releases, I've still only taken short turn-around trips on the Enterprise, and *Doctor Who* was nothing more than "silly

British stuff" preventing my grandmother from watching Orlando Wilson Fishing on PBS-- never mind the fact the show was on TBS and she could have watched it a few channels up.

I didn't realize what the disconnect I felt was for the first 13 years of my life or so, but in hindsight the goal was always to get out and find the place that I felt I belonged. I didn't know what I was running to or even what track I was running on (you'll find I love to stretch metaphors to the breaking point), but I knew that D-ville, or more specifically, the rural south itself, wasn't where I was supposed to be.

***

At the end of eighth grade we were required to pick our elective course for our freshman year of high school. It was the first academic choice I ever remember making. I remember Ms. O'Neal, the school counselor, coming to talk to our class one day about choosing the electives and how we should take it seriously and give it real thought because the electives that we chose in high school could end up shaping who we are and what we do. I went home that evening and thought about the options.

Despite always having a strange desire to be contrary to whatever was deemed as "normal", I decided that the elective that I chose should be something that would help me fit in. I looked at the list that night weighing the factors and trying to find the balance of something that I'd not absolutely despise, but meet that goal of finding some common ground.

Auto mechanics? That could be interesting. My father was an excellent mechanic and I had a little experience checking air pressure and pumping oil.

Musical Theatre

Junior Reserve Officer Training Corp? I mean it doesn't get much more "fitting in with the locals" than walking around with guns, wooden or not - though I couldn't really picture myself planning to take on "Ol' Saddam."

Woodworking? I mean, why not? I had seen Monster Squad several times at that point. Worst comes to worst I could steal some silver dinnerware and make bullets or carve out some stakes for when 'kicking wolfman in the nards' wasn't quite good enough.

The morning came to make our choice. I honestly don't remember what I was going to choose because the choice was taken away from me by those dreaded three words that had plagued me all throughout school.

"Line up alphabetically."

Now, if your last name is Adams, Baker, or Calrissian you are probably a little confused about why that moment would inspire such dread, but when your last name is Webb and the already limited choices are being made alphabetically, hearing that is instant defeat. This choice that Ms. O'Neal had just twenty-four hours ago called, "The biggest academic choice you've made so far" was now going to be decided by the equivalent to turning the bag upside down and risking a face full of processed cheese dust just in case there was one Cheeto left.

Finally, "Webb. Stephen Webb." My time had come. "Take a look at the form here and select which elective you'd like to take next year." If it weren't for Tommy Yan who was behind me, I could have taken all day to make the decision, but instead I had to look at the list and make a choice. Hopefully there would be something left that would meet my criteria which due to the last name situation had devolved to "not totally awful".

There were only two options left that weren't crossed out and marked as "FULL" in Ms. O'Neal's bubbly handwriting.

Home Economics.

Drama.

Neither of these were on my radar. Neither looked especially appealing to me, so I closed my eyes, flipped a mental coin and begrudgingly placed a checkmark next to "Drama".

✱✱✱

Ken Holder, or simply "Holder" as everyone lovingly referred to him, would eventually become my vocal coach, a father figure, a mentor, and friend. On that first day of high school however, he was my high school drama teacher. I remember walking into the drama room, the place that would become my "home base" for the next 4 years, and being cautiously intrigued. We were told to sit in the floor in a circle. There was a girl next to me who was too shy to even tell her name to the class, and she looked as if she would rather be anywhere but there. Her last name was Williams, so in all likelihood the Alphabetical Monster had struck again. Holder walked up to her and quietly said, "May I please see your hand?" The girl timidly opened up her hand, palm to the ceiling, and he took his pen and drew a tiny dot in the center of her palm and asked her to show it to the entire class.

We all had quizzical looks on our faces as he simultaneously explained the dot both to her and to the rest of the class. He had a real gift for making you feel like he was talking directly to you even though he was addressing a crowd. "That is your 'too wonderful' dot. I know today is scary and a lot to take in, but at any point you feel scared or lost, look at that dot and it will remind you that you are too wonderful not to be heard and seen. Too wonderful to not share your thoughts if you want." Ok, yeah, you might be thinking that it's a little cheesy and as the snarky adult sitting here writing this I can't argue that point - though I will say that maybe a little cheesy is exactly what we need to survive this world sometimes. That moment stuck with me and I decided right then and there that maybe this drama thing wasn't going to be so bad.

My freshman and sophomore years were great. I won't bore you with the details of one-act play competitions, improv studies and musical rehearsal 5-6 hours a day in addition to school. Let's just say Ms. O'Neal was right. The choice of Drama as my elective, regardless of how limited it may have seemed at the time, was not only the most important academic decision that I had made, but it has proven to be one of the most important decisions I've made to this day. If you believe in the butterfly effect, that day at the end of eighth grade was that linchpin moment that set all the other important decisions and framework of my life into motion. It was in that Drama Room where I discovered my first real fandom. Musical Theatre.

I became consumed with learning everything about Broadway that I could get my hands on and eventually I found IT, the most amazing musical that my mind could comprehend: Les Miserables.

Yeah, I said Les Mis. I bet you didn't see that coming given the title of this essay, right? Stick with me - it all ties together.

Over those first couple of years of high school I was lucky to have seen National Tour productions of musicals that came through Atlanta. Miss Saigon was my first "big theatre" experience and when that helicopter landed at the end of Act One my mind was blown. I remember being told, "It was even cooler on Broadway." Holder and my parents had worked together to organize a trip that would take me to New York City for the dream experience of seeing a Broadway Show. I was going to get to see Les Miserables live on stage. While I had performed many flawless performances of it in my bedroom, the ability to see this on stage wasn't something that happened daily to a kid in a blue collar, paycheck to paycheck household 895 miles from the Great White Way. For my 17-year-old self this was winning the lottery.

December 29th, 1996 - 1pm, Eastern Standard Time

It was a cold Wednesday in New York as I sauntered out of the Edison Hotel that afternoon with a bounce in my step, knowing that in just 7 short hours I was going to see my favorite show on Broadway. Of course that was the evening performance. We had tickets to a matinee that I had to "get through" before I could finally meet Marius, Eponine, and Valjean. Holder had wanted to see this new "rock musical" called RENT. By December of 1996 it had already won 4 Tonys, won the Pulitzer, and was the toast of the town. It was the kind of phenomenon that we hadn't seen before on Broadway and wouldn't see again until Hamilton came along nearly 20 years later. None of that mattered to me – I had my "know-it-all" blinders on and had pointedly avoided learning anything about this phenomenon, because it wasn't "Broadway enough." Maybe the best way to ensure that I will love something is to go into it with 'ambivalence with just a dash of reluctance.'

We took our seats for the performance and I remember the set looking shabby and unimpressive and there being a faint mist of smoke in the theatre. I didn't understand why this was so exciting to my mentor, but there was an undeniable buzz in the air.

Musical Theatre

I sat there, waiting for that moment when the lights go down and the orchestra starts playing, but that never came. Instead, the theatre stayed lit and a group of actors who didn't look that much older than me took the stage. One of them, wearing a maroon and periwinkle sweater stepped forward and said, "We begin on Christmas Eve…"

***

Two years earlier Holder had a bone marrow transplant and extensive treatments for leukemia. He was out of school the entire 2nd half of my freshman year and we would get generic updates about how "he's doing fine" and "he'll be back soon". I hoped for the best. I prayed to a God that I wasn't sure existed. I sent out "good juju" into the universe. But you never know if someone is going to win the battle when they are fighting for their life. He fought hard and he beat it. He came back, weaker and frailer on the outside, but with a renewed spirit of "I'm not going to let this beat me." He had adopted a mantra. "No Day But Today."

***

As the last chorus of "No Day But Today" filled the Nederlander that afternoon, I looked over at Holder who was crying through a look of absolute peaceful contentment. I realized I was doing the same.

December 29th, 1996 - 7pm, Eastern Standard Time

So yeah… *Les Mis*. I mean, sure – I enjoyed it… but I found myself sitting in the Imperial Theatre looking at the characters that had been the purpose of this trip just a mere 8 hours prior, but instead of focusing on them I was thinking about Collins, Angel, and Mimi's pants. (Blue vinyl skin tight pants weren't something I got to see often. Sue me.) As Marius was singing Empty

189

Chairs, my mind was on Mark Cohen, the narrator, who was so consumed with capturing the moments with his friends that he frequently found himself on the outside of them. Something about that really resonated with me. It all stuck with me for the next 4 months, which in teenage years is a lifetime. All I knew was that I wanted to go back to New York as quickly as possible and see this production again. Holder was happy to go again as chaperone, so I got a job working as a waiter in a coffee house on non-rehearsal nights and weekends so I could fund a trip back to New York over Spring Break just to see RENT again.

April 4th, 1996 - Afternoon, Eastern Standard Time

The day before Holder and I were scheduled to fly out to New York, this time with my then-girlfriend and her mother, he had a medical appointment. Holder was no stranger to those appointments after his battle with leukemia so I didn't think too much of it. Due to concerns about his immune system and cabin pressure, or some other issue that in hindsight I'm sure he was keeping from us, the Doctor advised him not to fly and to sit this trip out. We were disappointed, but he insisted that we all go and have a good time. He said that he looked forward to hearing all about it.

April 8th, 1997 - 7pm, Eastern Standard Time

We got to the theatre early and as I looked at the cast list I noticed that, for the second time, I was seeing the full cast except for Mark. Anthony Rapp, who originated the role, was caring for his mother as she battled cancer. He, understandably was missing the show a lot. I was already disappointed that I was going to see some understudy go on as Mark when an enthusiastic fan named Jo-Lin (who later became a friend), told me that this was also the understudy's first time going on in the role and the new Mimi's first performance as well as Tony Award Nominee (and Blue Vinyl Pants wearing) Daphne Rubin-Vega had just two nights prior been the first original cast member to leave the show. Great. My favorite character in the show, and I was seeing some dude do it for the first time. I pulled my understudy slip out of the Playbill and it read, "At this performance the role of Mark, usually played by Anthony Rapp, will be played by Norbert Leo Butz." Norbert Leo Butz? "Seriously, that's his name. This guy will never be anything!" Two Tony Awards later, I think Norbert is doing just fine.

That night the experience of watching the show touched me in a way that I still struggle to put into words. It was a theatre experience unlike any that I've ever had before and I never hope to have again. Angel, the "light and hope" of the group, dies in the 2nd Act of the show and under the best of circumstances it is heart wrenching - but on that night it wasn't Angel. It was my friend. My mentor. As I watched those characters cope with Angel getting ill and eventually dying I formed a bond with that show. I only remember a few specific details of the show itself, but I will never forget how I felt watching it. It was there in the that Mezzanine where I first really grasped the concept of how important it was for everyone to find a place they belong, but more importantly that you needed to hold on to it once you had it.

***

Less than two weeks later, back home in Georgia, I was at a Video Arcade trying to get my mind off of things. I hadn't been able to visit Holder because his condition had worsened. Due to his immune system being weak, the hospital would only allow family to visit him. In between the sounds of pinball machines and air hockey tables, I heard my mobile phone ring. I figured it was just my parents asking where I was and when I'd be home. It was my dad, but he didn't ask about my location and he didn't ask what time I'd be home. He was calling to tell me that a call had come in a few minutes earlier. Holder's body had rejected the bone marrow entirely and he was gone.

> ...the stars gleam/the poets dream/the eagles fly...
> Without You.

The next few months were full of teen angst. The cast recording of RENT got me through not only the loss of Holder, but in the span of about 6 months I also lost my grandfather, a friend who was the same age as me, and several of my girlfriend's close friends who had died tragically in a car accident. It was far more loss than anyone should have to deal with, but it's especially hard when it all occurs between Christmas and your high school graduation.

Eventually, playing the CD on my Discman stopped being as therapeutic and I needed to "change my meds." I found online communities like rec.arts.theatre.musicals.Rent and CliqueyBitches where I made connections with people who also loved the show as passionately as I did. It was there that I made a discovery that changed me. It turns out that people would sneak tape recorders into the show and record the performances onto cassettes. Bootlegs!

I became obsessed with trading bootlegs of different performances of *RENT*. Different understudies, cast combinations, etc. This was before you could simply upload/download media clips online so you'd have to make a copy of your tape and mail it to people who would make copies of their tapes for you. This turned into an obsession. I wanted to own every show and hear everyone I could in every role. It distracted me from the fact that my running away was being done on a treadmill.

July 1st, 1997 - 8pm, Pacific Standard Time

The 2nd National Tour of Rent was opening at the La Jolla Playhouse just outside of San Diego. They had announced a cast that featured Wilson Cruz from *My So Called Life* playing Angel and Neil Patrick Harris, who at that time was known almost exclusively for *Doogie Howser M.D.,* playing Mark. Before the show even took place I was trying to ensure I'd get recordings of that First Preview as quickly as possible. I found someone online who was not only going, but had a friend who was going to record it. I badgered her for days after the performance asking "What do I have to trade?" "How much money would you need etc.?" Finally, I think I had bored her and she passed me off to her friend, the one with the recorder, to continue our AOL IM chat. I learned later that the exact words were, "Talk to this guy, I'm bored." The friend and I hit it off extremely well and continued talking long after the tapes were traded.

Her name was Anji and I was definitely smitten. It was the first time I remember feeling much of anything after the months of grieving that I had been going though. I mean, she lived in California and I lived in Georgia so I never thought it could develop into anything. This was well before swiping right was how you found a mate on the internet. In 1997 the protocol was "don't date online, you'll die." Still, I liked her a lot.

In December of that year, the show had moved to Los Angeles and I decided a visit had to happen. I didn't have a ton of money, so I arranged to stay with Anji. I was nervous and excited. She picked me up at the airport and it was like one of those cavity-inducing movie moments where the world slows down and the object of your desire starts going down the stairs very slowly while *Sixpence None The Richer* suddenly starts crooning about kissing. We hit it off in person just as well as we did online and I dare say it was love at first sight. I mean – it had to be, this entire experience was bound together by musicals right?

This was the first time I would be seeing *RENT* since April. It would also be the first time I was seeing it from the Front Row which aided you in feeling like you were part of the show. That Los Angeles performance on December 16th, 1997 was the release of all the emotion that had been building since it started in April in New York. Mark Leroy Jackson's "I'll Cover You (Reprise)" served not only as Collins' goodbye to Angel, but there in the Ahmanson Theatre it served as my long overdue goodbye to Ken Holder.

Anji and I spent an amazing week together, yet we both were coming at this with a fair amount of caution because we knew that this wonderful musical relationship was well into the second act and the 11 o'clock number was almost here.

December 23rd, 1997 - 10pm, Pacific Standard Time

I was devastated as my plane left LAX. I had just had closure from one type of loss and now here I was experiencing it again in a completely different, yet equally brutal, form. That long redeye home was horrible, and that was just for the lady who had a sobbing 18 year old beside her on the plane.

Musical Theatre

For the next week, I moped around my house wearing headphones listening to the tape that we had recorded on my Walkman of that performance of *RENT*. Despite listening over and over to the message of this show for nearly a year, I finally heard it for the first time.

"There's only now, there's only here

Give in to love, or live in fear

No other path, No other way

No day but today"

I never felt like Georgia was where I belonged, yet I had let the last year confine me. The fear of losing other people, or failing, had kept me grounded in one spot. I started to feel like I was a hypocrite if I didn't "give into love". I had been trying to escape my life. All the way to Los Angeles and back, I was trying to run away from what I knew, but I was going about it all wrong. Running away from something only really works if you're also running towards something in the process.

December 29th, 1997 - 1:36pm, Eastern Standard Time

I can't believe a year went by so fast.

Exactly one year, (well 525,636 minutes) after I sat down in the Nederlander Theatre to watch *RENT* for the first time, I stepped onto on a Greyhound Bus bound for Los Angeles with a single bag full of my past and a blank slate for my future. Anji and I were going to get our "happily ever after" at the end of this crazy tale.

This is where the musical ends most of the time, right? The boy and the girl, despite all the odds, find a way to be together. We rarely find out what they actually do with that chance.

Stephen Webb

Today - Now, Universal Time

Well – the speedy Cliff's Notes version is this – I've been with Anji, who in short order became Anji Webb, for 20 years. In 2008, we went to the closing performance of RENT on Broadway. We experienced the show that brought us together one last time, but this time it was special for a different reason because she was 7 months pregnant with our son Cooper – who I swear to you, was kicking and bopping along during "La Vie Boheme". It was important for us to experience the show that brought us together as a family.

For all of us in the *RENT* scene in the late 90s, it was never just about the show. It was about the friendships formed from the experience of "the line". We were a group of people who all had our own stories of loss, love, and connection with this material. A group who each had their individual experience of dealings with things like life and death through a different filter because of where we were and what we loved. We were a group of people who didn't always feel that we fit in individually, but we worked as a cohesive unit that had that our love for the show in common.

That is the essence of fandom for me. Finding people who understand why you are so crazy about something that the vast majority of society views as "not that big of a deal". It isn't crazy for us. It is love and marriage, it is counseling and mourning. It is creation, and above all else – it is life.

ABOUT THE CONTRIBUTORS

Dr. Melissa D. Aaron teaches at Cal Poly Pomona, and specializes in Renaissance drama and werewolves in Harry Potter. Pinkie Pie is Best Pony.

Emma Caywood is a Children's and Youth Librarian in Wellesley, MA, where she recommends geeky books, geekily entertains babies, hosts geeky ukulele jam sessions, and turns picture books into geeky plays. She has previously worked as a drama teacher, storyteller, actress, environmental science teacher, playwright, literary manager for screenwriters, grammar teacher, mask maker, and once did a one day stint as a the receptionist at the Jazzercise Corporate Headquarters.

Clay Dockery is the co-head organizer of MISTI-Con a Harry Potter fan convention, co-founder and treasurer of Coal Hill, Inc., and Program & Education Director for the Interfaith Community a non-profit organization focused on helping families from different religious traditions authentically and respectfully navigate their challenges.

Will Dockery is a poet and singer/songwriter based in Columbus, GA.

Jennifer Drucker works as a graphic designer and fine artist. She loves to create many of the graphics, props and visuals for MISTI-Con, HP-NYC, and her Etsy shop, Jenny's Oubliette. In true Hufflepuff pride, she runs her own cake decorating business, Jenny's Cakes With Character, specializing in geek-themed culinary creations. Jennifer recently co-founded a fandom based party planning business, Geek Party Chic. She is happy to make life more beautiful, and edible too!

About The Contributors

Christine Evans is a performer, costumer, and cosplayer. She is the founder and costumer of C&C Costume factory which is dedicated to creating the highest quality costume experiences for everyone.

Dawn Ferchak is a lifelong fangirl. When not opining on her favorite fandoms, she can be found working as a professional writer and editor, planning new burlesque routines under her alter ego Regina Monologue, and helping animals as a rescue and rehabilitation volunteer. Read more of her Supernatural opinions at www.pieandshotguns.com.

Alex Fitzgerald is a student in Northern Virginia and lives with his wonderful girlfriend, Lauren.

Hannah Harkness is a stand-up comic, storyteller, and writer from Philadelphia, PA. She also hosts the most incompetent "let's play" gaming series on YouTube, Haneurysm.

Dustin Hausner has been a fan of comic books and science fiction for over 20 years. He has a Master's in Negotiation and Conflict Resolution from Columbia University.

Erik Henriksen is basically Catbert – an Evil Director of Human Resources – but otherwise decent human being with an overactive imagination and overinflated sense of self-importance. He is an avid tabletop gamer who invests a silly amount of time creating psychically damaged characters to play out painfully obvious inadequacies to a bored audience of fellow players. He watches enough television to disprove the myth that watching too much TV makes you go blind.

Andy Hicks is a radio and TV producer in Boston. He is also the Vice President of Coal Hill Inc. and writes and performs the "Epic Rap Battles of Who-Story". Occasionally he sleeps.

About The Contributors

Scarlett Jaye is a freelance writer, amateur seamstress, and cosplayer who considers herself "just a kid from Brooklyn". She is a proud New Yorker in part because so many of her favorite fictional heroes, from Captain America to Spider Man, all hail from the Big Apple.

Terry Molloy took over the role of Dalek creator Davros in Doctor Who's "Resurrection of the Daleks," reprising the role in two subsequent stories, as well as appearing as a policeman in "Attack of of the Cybermen". In recent years, Molloy has reprised the role of Davros in the Big Finish Productions audio dramas Davros, The Juggernauts, Terror Firma, Masters of War, The Davros Mission and the four-part miniseries I, Davros, as well as in a 2005 stage production, The Trial of Davros. Terry also took over the role of Stan Harvey in the ITV soap opera Crossroads, has appeared on BBC 7 opposite the late Nicholas Courtney in The Scarifyers audio series, and more recently in BBC Radio 4's The Archers.

Amanda-Rae Prescott is an avid live tweeter, blogger, and cosplayer of period dramas. When she is not crying over how unfair *The Halcyon's* cancellation was, she is the Director of Cosplay Programming and Press Liaison for L.I. Who.

Betsy R. Shepherd is a lawyer in the Atlanta, GA area. In addition to baseball, she loves a good space opera and an occasional game of Dungeons & Dragons.

Julia Siciliano is, like fan-fiction, an amalgamation of all those things the author wishes she could be and were possible.

Cat Smith is an actor, musician, writer, costume geek and mom, in any order you like. She performs at conventions throughout the country as Miss Nerdstiles. Give her enough ukuleles, and she'll save the world.

About The Contributors

Robert Smith? is the author of *Who is the Doctor, Who's 50 and The Doctor's Are In* (ECW Press), guides to the wonderful world of Doctor Who. He's also the editor extraordinaire of the *Outside In* series of pop culture reviews with a twist (ATB Publishing), covering Doctor Who, Star Trek and Buffy. In his day job, he's a professor of mathematics and a world leading expert on zombies. Really.

Stephen Webb is a SAHD, husband, podcaster, writer, performer, and all around geek. He is the President of Coal Hill Inc., a non-profit organization dedicated to enhancing fandom by creating fun and innovative podcasts, 'music, art, and interactive experiences.

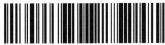

Made in the USA
Middletown, DE
16 January 2018